Study Guide to accompany

The Human Body in Health & Disease

Fourth Edition

Linda Swisher, RN, EdD

ELSEVIER
MOSBY

ELSEVIER
MOSBY
11830 Westline Industrial Drive
St. Louis, MO 63146

Study Guide to accompany The Human Body
in Health & Disease, FOURTH EDITION

Previous editions copyrighted 2002, 1997, 1992.

ISBN-13: 978-0-323-03644-3
ISBN-10: 0-323-03644-9

Senior Acquisitions Editor: Tom Wilhelm
Managing Editor: Jeff Downing
Developmental Editor: Jennifer Anderson
Publishing Services Manager: Deborah L. Vogel
Senior Project Manager: Ann E. Rogers
Senior Book Designer: Julia Dummitt

Printed in the United States of America

Last digit is the print number: 9 8 7 6 5 4 3

Acknowledgments

I wish to express my appreciation to the staff of Mosby, Inc., especially Tom Wilhelm, Jeff Downing, and Jennifer Anderson for opening the door and assisting me with this text. My continued admiration and gratitude to Gary Thibodeau and Kevin Patton for an outstanding text. Your time and dedication to science education will, hopefully, inspire potential caregivers and improve the quality of health care for the future.

To my family, Brian, friends and colleagues, my thanks for your assistance and support.

To Bill, the angel on my shoulder, I feel your presence, love, and guidance always.

Finally, to the designer of the human body, this book is dedicated. What a miraculous creation!

Linda Swisher, RN, EdD

Preface

TO THE INSTRUCTOR

This Study Guide is designed to help your students master basic anatomy and physiology. It works in two ways.

First, the section of the preface titled "To the Student," contains detailed instructions on:

- How to achieve good grades in anatomy and physiology
- How to read the textbook
- How to use the exercises in this Study Guide
- How to use visual memory as a learning tool
- How to use mnemonic devices as learning aids
- How to prepare for an examination
- How to take an examination
- How to find out why questions were missed on an examination

Second, the Study Guide itself contains features that facilitate learning. These features include the following:

1. LEARNING OBJECTIVES, designed to break down the process of learning into small units. The questions in this Study Guide have been developed to help the student master the learning objectives identified at the beginning of each chapter in the text. The Guide is also sequenced to correspond to key areas of each chapter. A variety of questions have been prepared to cover the material effectively and expose the student to multiple learning approaches.

2. CROSSWORD PUZZLES, to encourage the use of new vocabulary words and emphasize the proper spelling of these terms.

3. OPTIONAL APPLICATION QUESTIONS, particularly targeted for the health occupations student, but appropriate for any student of anatomy and physiology because questions are based entirely on information contained within the chapter.

4. DIAGRAMS, with key features marked by numbers for identification. Students can easily check their work by comparing the diagram in the workbook with the equivalent figure in the text.

5. PAGE NUMBER REFERENCES, in the answer sections. Each answer is keyed to the appropriate text page. Additionally, questions are grouped into specific topics that correspond to the text. Each major topic of the Study Guide provides references to specific areas of the text, so that students having difficulty with a particular grouping of questions have a specific reference area to assist them with remedial work. This is of great assistance to both instructor and student, because remedial work is made easier and more effective when the area of weakness is identified accurately.

These features should make mastery of the material a rewarding experience for both instructor and student.

TO THE STUDENT

How to Achieve Good Grades in Anatomy and Physiology

This Study Guide is designed to help you be successful in learning anatomy and physiology. Before you begin using the Study Guide, read the following suggestions. Successful students understand effective study techniques and have good study habits.

How to Read the Textbook

Keep up with the reading assignments. Read the textbook assignment before the instructor covers the material in a lecture. If you have failed to read the assignment beforehand, you will not grasp what the instructor is talking about in the lecture. When you read, do the following:

1. As you finish reading a sentence, ask yourself if you understand it. If you do not, put a question mark in the margin by that sentence. If the instructor does not clarify the material in lecture, ask him or her to further explain it to you.

2. Do the learning objectives in the text. A learning objective is a specific task that you are expected to be able to do after you have read a chapter. It sets specific goals for the student and breaks down learning into small units. It emphasizes the key points that the author is making in the chapter.

3. Underline and make notes in the margin to highlight key ideas, mark something you need to reinforce at a later time, or indicate things that you do not understand.

4. If you come to a word you do not understand, look it up in a dictionary. Write the word on one side of an index card and its definition on the other side. Carry these cards with you, and when you have a spare minute, use them like flash cards. If you do not know how to spell or pronounce a word, you will have a hard time remembering it.

5. Carefully study each diagram and illustration as you read. Many students ignore these aids. The author included them to help students understand the material.

6. Summarize what you read. After finishing a paragraph, try to restate the main ideas. Do this again when you finish the chapter. Identify and review in your mind the main concepts of the chapter. Check to see if you are correct. In short, be an active reader. Do not just stare at a page or read it superficially.

7. Finally, attack each unit of learning with a positive mental attitude. Motivation and perseverance are prime factors in achieving successful grades. The combination of your instructor, the text, the Study Guide, and your dedicated work will lead to success for you in anatomy and physiology.

How to Use the Exercises in this Study Guide

After you have read a chapter and learned all the new words, begin working with the Study Guide. Read the overview of the chapter, which summarizes the main points.

Familiarize yourself with the "Topics for Review" section, which emphasizes the learning objectives outlined in the text. Complete the questions and diagrams in the Study Guide. The questions are sequenced to follow the chapter outline and headings and are divided into small sections to facilitate learning. A variety of questions are offered throughout the Study Guide to help you cover the material effectively. The following examples are among the exercises that have been included to assist you.

Multiple Choice Questions

Multiple choice questions will have only one correct answer for you to select from the several possibilities presented. There are two types of multiple choice questions that you need to be acquainted with:

1. "None of the above is correct" questions. These questions test your ability to recall rather than recognize the correct answer. You would select the "none of the above" choice only if all the other choices in that particular question were incorrect.

2. Sequence questions. These questions test your ability to arrange a list of structures in the correct order. In this type of question, you are asked to determine the sequence of the structures given in the various

choices, and then you are to select the structure listed that would be third in that sequence, as in this example.

Which one of the following structures is the third through which food passes?
A. Stomach
B. Mouth
C. Large intestine
D. Esophagus
E. Anus

The correct answer is *A*.

Matching Questions

Matching questions ask the student to select the correct answer from a list of terms and to write that answer in the space provided.

True or False Questions

True or false questions ask you to write "T" in the answer space if you agree with that statement. If you disagree with the statement, you will circle the incorrect word(s) and write the correct word(s) in the answer space.

Identify the Term that Does Not Belong

In questions that ask you to identify the incorrect term, three words are given that relate to each other in structure or function, and one more word is included that has no relationship, or has an opposing relationship to the other three terms. You are asked to circle the term that does not relate to the others. An example might be: iris, cornea, stapes, retina. You would circle the word *stapes* because all other terms refer to the eye.

Fill-in-the-Blank Questions

Fill-in-the-blank questions ask you to recall missing word(s) and insert it (them) into the answer blank(s). These questions may involve sentences or paragraphs.

Application Questions

Application questions ask you to make judgments about a situation based on the information in the chapter. These questions may ask you how you would respond to a situation or to suggest a possible diagnosis for a set of symptoms.

Charts

Several charts have been included that correspond to figures in the text. Areas have been omitted so that you can fill them in and test your recall of these important areas.

Word Finds

The Study Guide includes word find puzzles that allow you to identify key terms in the chapter in an interesting and challenging way.

Crossword Puzzles

Vocabulary words from the "New Words" section at the end of each chapter of the text have been developed into crossword puzzles. This encourages recall and proper spelling. Occasionally, an exercise uses scrambled words to encourage recall and spelling.

Labeling Exercises

Labeling exercises present diagrams with parts that are not identified. For each of these diagrams, you are to print the name of each numbered part on the appropriately numbered line. You may choose to further distinguish the structures by coloring them with a variety of colors. After you have written down the names of the structures to be identified, check your answers. When it comes time to review for an examination you can place a sheet of paper over your answers to test yourself.

After completing the exercises in the Study Guide, check your answers. If they are not correct, refer to the page listed with the answer, and review it for further clarification. If you still do not understand the question or the answer, ask your instructor for further explanation or assistance.

If you have difficulty with several questions from one section, refer to the pages given at the end of the section. After reviewing the section, try to answer the questions again. If you are still having difficulty, talk to your instructor.

How to Use Visual Memory

Visual memory is another important tool in learning. If I asked you to picture an elephant in your mind, with all its external parts labeled, you could do that easily. Visual memory is a powerful key to learning. Whenever possible, try to build a memory picture. Remember, a picture is worth a thousand words.

Visual memory works especially well with the sequencing of items, such as circulatory pathways and the passage of air or food. Students who try to learn sequencing by memorizing a list of words do poorly on examinations. If they forget one word in the sequence, they then may forget the remaining words as well. With a memory picture you can pick out the important features.

How to Use Mnemonic Devices

Mnemonic devices are little jingles that you memorize to help you remember things. If you make up your own, they will stick with you longer. Here are three examples of such devices:

"On Old Olympus' towering tops a Finn and German viewed some hops." This one is used to remember the cranial nerves. Each word begins with the same letter as does the name of one of the nerves.

"C. Hopkins CaFe where they serve Mg NaCl." This mnemonic device reminds you of the chemical symbols for the biologically important electrolytes.

"Roy G. Biv." This mnemonic device helps you remember the colors of the visible light spectrum.

How to Prepare for an Examination

Prepare far in advance for an examination. Actually, your preparation for an examination should begin on the first day of class. Keeping up with your assignments daily makes the final preparation for an examination much easier. You should begin your final preparation at least three nights before the test. Last-minute studying usually means poor results and limited retention.

1. Make sure that you understand and can answer all of the learning objectives for the chapter on which you are being tested.

2. Review the appropriate questions in this Study Guide. Review is something that you should do after every class and at the end of every study session. It is important to keep going over the material until you have a thorough understanding of the chapter and rapid recall of its contents. If review becomes a daily habit, studying for the actual examination will not be difficult. Go through each question and write down an answer. Do the same with the labeling of each structure on the appropriate diagrams. If you have al-

ready done this as part of your daily review, cover the answers with a piece of paper and quiz yourself again.

3. Check the answers that you have written down against the correct answers in the back of the Study Guide. Go back and study the areas in the text that refer to questions that you missed and then try to answer those questions again. If you still cannot answer a question or label a structure correctly, ask your instructor for help.

4. As you read a chapter, ask yourself what questions you would ask if you were writing a test on that unit. You will most likely ask yourself many of the questions that will show up on your examinations.

5. Get a good night's sleep before the test. Staying up late and upsetting your biorhythms will only make you less efficient during the test.

How to Take an Examination

The Day of the Test

1. Get up early enough to avoid rushing. Eat appropriately. Your body needs fuel, but a heavy meal just before a test is not a good idea.

2. Keep calm. Briefly look over your notes. If you have prepared for the test properly, there will be no need for last-minute cramming.

3. Make certain that you have everything you need for the test: pens, pencils, test sheets, and so forth.

4. Allow enough time to get to the examination site. Missing your bus, getting stuck in traffic, or being unable to find a parking space will not put you in a good frame of mind to do well on the examination.

During the Examination

1. Pay careful attention to the instructions for the test.

2. Note any corrections.

3. Budget your time so that you will be able to finish the test.

4. Ask the instructor for clarification if you do not understand a question or an instruction.

5. Concentrate on your own test paper and do not allow yourself to be distracted by others in the room.

Hints for Taking a Multiple Choice Test

1. Read each question carefully. Pay attention to each word.

2. Cross out obviously wrong choices and think about those that are left.

3. Go through the test once, quickly answering the questions you are sure of; then go back over the test and answer the rest of the questions.

4. Fill in the answer spaces completely and make your marks heavy. Erase answers completely if you make a mistake.

5. If you must guess, stick with your first hunch. Most often, students will change right answers to wrong ones.

6. If you will not be penalized for guessing, do not leave any blanks.

Hints for Taking an Essay Test

1.   Budget time for each question.

2.   Write legibly and try to spell words correctly.

3.   Be concise, complete, and specific. Do not be repetitious or long-winded.

4.   Organize your answer in an outline—this helps not only the student but also the person who grades the test.

5.   Answer each question as thoroughly as you can, but leave some room for possible additions.

Hints for Taking a Laboratory Practical Examination

Students have a hard time with this kind of test. Visual memory is very important here. To put it simply, you must be able to identify every structure you have studied. If you are unable to identify a structure, then you will be unable to answer any questions about that structure.

Possible questions that could appear on an examination of this type might include:

1.   Identification of a structure, organ, or feature.

2.   Identification of the function of a structure, organ, or feature.

3.   Sequence questions for air flow, passage of food, urine, and so forth.

4.   Disease questions (for example, if an organ fails, what disease will result?).

How to Find Out Why Questions Were Missed on an Examination

After the Examination

Go over your test after it has been scored to see what you missed and why you missed it. You can pick up important clues that will help you on future examinations. Ask yourself these questions:

1.   Did I miss questions because I did not read them carefully?

2.   Did I miss questions because I had gaps in my knowledge?

3.   Did I miss questions because I could not determine scientific words?

4.   Did I miss questions because I did not have good visual memory of things?

Be sure to go back and learn the things you did not know. Chances are these topics will come up on the final examination.

Your grades in other classes will improve as well when you apply these study methods. Learning should be fun. With these helpful hints and this Study Guide you should be able to achieve the grades you desire. Good luck!

Contents

CHAPTER 1

An Introduction to the Structure and Function of the Body

A command of terminology is necessary for a student to be successful in any area of science. This chapter defines the terminology and concepts that are basic to the field of anatomy and physiology. Building a firm foundation in these language skills will assist you with all future chapters.

The study of anatomy and physiology involves the structure and function of an organism and the relationship of its parts. It begins with a basic organization of the body into different structural levels. Beginning with the smallest level (the cell) and progressing to the largest, most complex level (the system), this chapter familiarizes you with the terminology and the levels of organization needed to facilitate the study of the body as a part or as a whole.

It is also important to be able to identify and describe specific body areas or regions as we progress in this field. The anatomical position is used as a reference position when dissecting the body into planes, regions, or cavities. The terminology defined in this chapter allows you to describe the areas efficiently and accurately.

Finally, the process of homeostasis is reviewed. This state of relative constancy in the chemical composition of body fluids is necessary for good health. In fact, the very survival of the body depends on the successful maintenance of homeostasis.

TOPICS FOR REVIEW

Before progressing to Chapter 2, you should have an understanding of the structural levels of organization; the planes, regions, and cavities of the body; the terminology used to describe these areas; and the concept of homeostasis as it relates to the survival of the species.

STRUCTURAL LEVELS OF ORGANIZATION

Match the term on the left with the proper selection on the right.

_____ 1. Organism   A. Many similar cells that act together to perform a common function

_____ 2. Cells   B. The most complex units that make up the body

_____ 3. Tissue   C. A group of several different kinds of tissues arranged to perform a special function

_____ 4. Organ   D. Denotes a living thing

_____ 5. Systems   E. The smallest "living" units of structure and function in the body

▷ *If you have had difficulty with this section, review pages 1-4.*

ANATOMICAL POSITION

Match the term on the left with the proper selection on the right.

_____ 6. Body

_____ 7. Arms

_____ 8. Feet

_____ 9. Prone

_____ 10. Supine

A. At the sides

B. Face upward

C. Erect

D. Face downward

E. Forward

▶ *If you have had difficulty with this section, review page 4.*

ANATOMICAL DIRECTIONS

Planes or Body Sections

Fill in the crossword puzzle.

ACROSS
12. Lower or below
13. Horizontal plane
16. Toward the midline of the body

DOWN
11. Upper or above
14. Front (abdominal side)
15. Toward the side of the body
17. Farthest from the point of origin of a body point

Circle the correct answer.

18. The stomach is (superior or inferior) to the diaphragm.

19. The nose is located on the (anterior or posterior) surface of the body.

20. The lungs lie (medial or lateral) to the heart.

21. The elbow lies (proximal or distal) to the forearm.

22. The skin is (superficial or deep) to the muscles below it.

23. A midsagittal plane divides the body into (equal or unequal) parts.

24. A frontal plane divides the body into (anterior and posterior or superior and inferior) sections.

25. A transverse plane divides the body into (right and left or upper and lower) sections.

26. A coronal plane may also be referred to as a (sagittal or frontal) plane.

▷ *If you have had difficulty with this section, review pages 4-6.*

BODY CAVITIES

Select the correct term from the choices given and insert the letter in the answer blank.

A. Ventral cavity   B. Dorsal cavity

_____ 27. Thoracic

_____ 28. Cranial

_____ 29. Abdominal

_____ 30. Pelvic

_____ 31. Mediastinum

_____ 32. Spinal

_____ 33. Pleural

▷ *If you have had difficulty with this section, review pages 6-8.*

BODY REGIONS

Circle the one that does not belong.

34. Axial   Head   Trunk   Extremities

35. Axillary   Cephalic   Brachial   Antecubital

36. Frontal   Orbital   Plantar   Nasal

37. Carpal   Crural   Plantar   Pedal

38. Cranial   Occipital   Tarsal   Temporal

▷ *If you have had difficulty with this section, review pages 8-10.*

If the following statement is true, insert "T" in the answer blank. If the statement is false, circle the incorrect word(s) and insert the correct word(s) in the answer blank.

_____ 39. The term *autopsy* comes from the Greek words auto (self) and opsis (view).

_____ 40. Autopsies are usually performed in four stages.

_____ 41. In the first stage of an autopsy, the exterior of the body is examined for abnormalities such as wounds or scars.

_____ 42. The face, arms, and legs are usually dissected during the second stage of an autopsy.

_____ 43. Microscopic examination of tissues occurs during all stages of an autopsy.

_____ 44. Tests to analyze the chemical content of body fluids or to determine the presence of infectious organisms may also be performed during an autopsy.

▶ *If you have had difficulty with this section, review page 7.*

THE BALANCE OF BODY FUNCTIONS

Fill in the blanks.

45. _____ depends on the body's ability to maintain or restore homeostasis.

46. *Homeostasis* is the term used to describe the relative constancy of the body's
_____.

47. During exercise, homeostasis is disrupted and body CO_2 levels _____.

48. Changes and functions that occur during the early years are called _____.

49. Changes and functions that occur after young adulthood are called _____.

50. Homeostatic control mechanisms are categorized as either _____ or
_____ feedback loops.

51. Negative feedback loops are _____ mechanisms.

52. Positive feedback control loops are _____.

▶ *If you have had difficulty with this section, review pages 10-15.*

APPLYING WHAT YOU KNOW

53. Mrs. Hunt has had an appendectomy. The nurse is preparing to change the dressing. She knows that the appendix is located in the right iliac inguinal region, the distal portion extending at an angle into the hypogastric region. Place an X on the diagram where the nurse will place the dressing.

54. Mrs. Wiedeke noticed a lump in her breast. Dr. Reeder noted on her chart that a small mass was located in the left breast medial to the nipple. Place an X where Mrs. Wiedeke's lump would be located.

55. Heather was injured in a bicycle accident. X-ray films revealed that she had a fracture of the right patella. A cast was applied beginning at the distal femoral region and extending to the pedal region. Place an X where Heather's cast begins and ends.

56. Word Find

Can you find the 18 terms from this chapter that are listed below? Words may be spelled top to bottom, bottom to top, right to left, left to right, or diagonally.

Anatomy   Posterior
Atrophy   Proximal
Homeostasis   Sagittal
Medial   Superficial
Mediastinum   Superior
Organ   System
Organization   Thoracic
Physiology   Tissue
Pleural   Ventral

```
N  H  L  T  E  B  W  N  G  N  M  M  Y  X  A
O  O  H  A  V  U  U  C  L  W  E  P  N  G  L
I  M  U  N  I  T  S  A  I  D  E  M  W  A  L
T  E  R  T  V  C  T  S  I  C  J  S  R  T  K
A  O  N  O  P  T  I  A  I  W  A  T  Y  R  H
Z  S  Q  S  I  R  L  F  A  T  N  R  G  O  W
I  T  W  G  P  R  O  I  R  E  T  S  O  P  F
N  A  A  Z  J  E  E  X  V  E  E  H  L  H  Z
A  S  N  L  M  C  T  P  I  C  P  D  O  Y  T
G  I  C  A  Y  U  O  X  U  M  N  U  I  V  P
R  S  M  R  T  N  U  K  B  S  A  Y  S  V  M
O  R  C  U  R  O  I  R  B  S  Q  L  Y  U  G
L  H  X  E  M  P  M  E  T  S  Y  S  H  V  S
U  W  L  L  Q  D  U  Y  Y  N  E  E  P  J  B
Q  N  Z  P  K  D  B  O  D  C  G  I  N  J  A
```

DID YOU KNOW?

Many animals produce tears but only humans weep as a result of emotional stress.

CHECK YOUR KNOWLEDGE

Multiple Choice

Circle the correct answer.

1. The body's ability to respond continuously to changes in the environment and maintain consistency in the internal environment is called:
   A. Homeostasis
   B. Superficial
   C. Structural levels
   D. None of the above

2. The regions frequently used by health professionals to locate pain or tumors divides the abdomen into four basic areas called:
   A. Planes
   B. Cavities
   C. Pleural
   D. Quadrants

3. Which of the following organs or structures does *not* lie within the mediastinum?
   A. Aorta
   B. Liver
   C. Esophagus
   D. Trachea

4. A lengthwise plane running from front to back that divides the body into right and left sides is called:
   A. Transverse
   B. Coronal
   C. Frontal
   D. Sagittal

5. A study of the functions of living organisms and their parts is called:
   A. Physiology
   B. Chemistry
   C. Biology
   D. None of the above

6. The thoracic portion of the ventral body cavity is separated from the abdominopelvic portion by a muscle called the:
   A. Latissimus dorsi
   B. Rectus femoris
   C. Diaphragm
   D. Pectoralis

7. An organization of varying numbers and kinds of organs arranged together to perform a complex function is called a:
   A. Cell
   B. Tissue
   C. System
   D. Region

8. The plane that divides superior from inferior is known as the _____ plane.
   A. Transverse
   B. Sagittal
   C. Frontal
   D. None of the above

9. Which of the following structures does *not* lie within the abdominal cavity?
   A. Spleen
   B. Most of the small intestine
   C. Urinary bladder
   D. Stomach

10. Which of the following is an example of an upper abdominal region?
    A. Right iliac region
    B. Left hypochondriac region
    C. Left lumbar region
    D. Hypogastric region

11. The dorsal body cavity contains components of the:
    A. Reproductive system
    B. Digestive system
    C. Respiratory system
    D. Nervous system

12. What organ is *not* found in the pelvic cavity?
    A. Bladder
    B. Stomach
    C. Rectum
    D. Colon

13. Similar cells acting together to perform a common function exist at a level of organization called a/an:
    A. Organ
    B. Chemical
    C. Tissue
    D. System

14. Which of the following planes would be considered coronal?
    A. A plane that divides the body into anterior and posterior portions
    B. A plane that divides the body into upper and lower portions
    C. A plane that divides the body into right and left sides
    D. A plane that divides the body into superficial and deep portions

15. If your reference point is "nearest the trunk of the body" vs. "farthest from the trunk of the body," where does the elbow lie in relation to the wrist?
    A. Anterior
    B. Posterior
    C. Distal
    D. Proximal

16. In the anatomical position:
    A. The dorsal body cavity is anterior to the ventral
    B. Palms face toward the back of the body
    C. The body is erect
    D. All of the above

17. The buttocks are often used as intramuscular injection sites. This region can be called:
    A. Sacral
    B. Buccal
    C. Cutaneous
    D. Gluteal

18. In the human body, the chest region:
    A. Can be referred to as the thoracic cavity
    B. Is a component of the ventral body cavity
    C. Contains the mediastinum
    D. All of the above

19. Which of the following is *not* a component of the axial subdivision of the body?
    A. Upper extremity
    B. Neck
    C. Trunk
    D. Head

20. A synonym for medial is:
    A. Toward the side
    B. In front of
    C. Midline
    D. Anterior

Matching

Select the most appropriate answer in column B for each item in column A. (Only one answer is correct.)

Column A

_____ 21. Ventral

_____ 22. Skin

_____ 23. Transverse

_____ 24. Anatomy

_____ 25. Superficial

_____ 26. Pleural

_____ 27. Appendicular

_____ 28. Posterior

_____ 29. Midsagittal

_____ 30. System

Column B

A. Equal

B. Cutaneous

C. Lung

D. Extremities

E. Respiratory

F. Anterior

G. Structure

H. Surface

I. Back

J. Horizontal

Fill in the Blanks

Complete these statements.

31. A systemic approach to discovery is known as the _____.

32. A tentative explanation in research is known as a _____.

33. The testing of a hypothesis is_____.

34. A group getting a drug is the _____.

35. A group getting a substitute is the _____.

DORSAL AND VENTRAL BODY CAVITIES

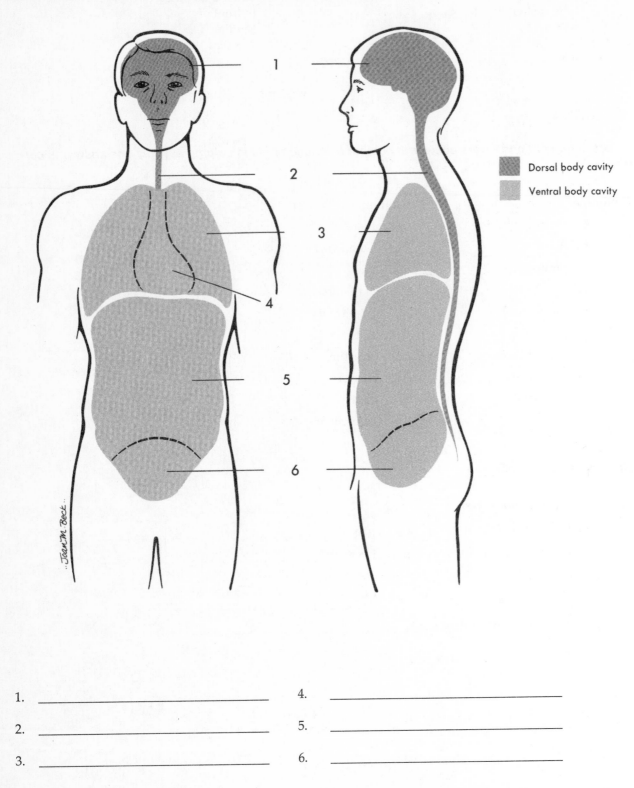

Dorsal body cavity
Ventral body cavity

1. _____   4. _____

2. _____   5. _____

3. _____   6. _____

DIRECTIONS AND PLANES OF THE BODY

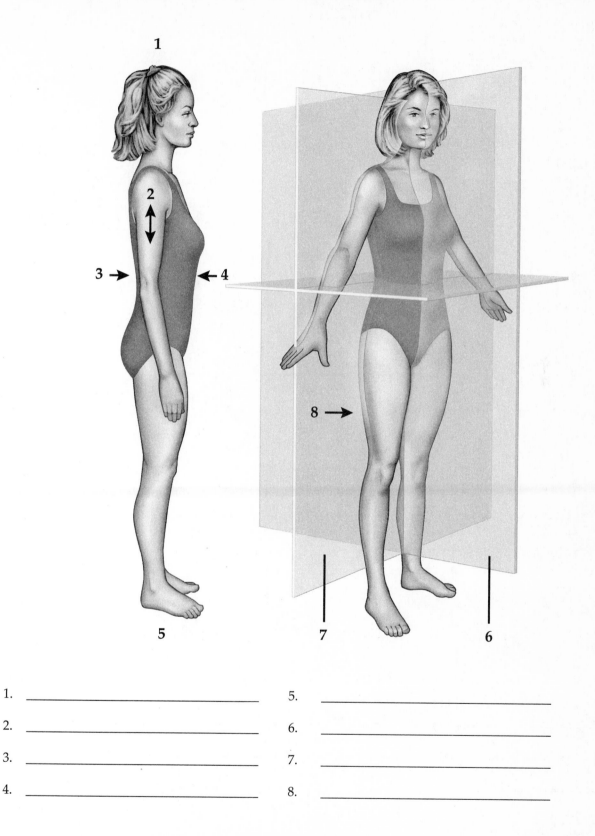

1. _____
2. _____
3. _____
4. _____

5. _____
6. _____
7. _____
8. _____

REGIONS OF THE ABDOMEN

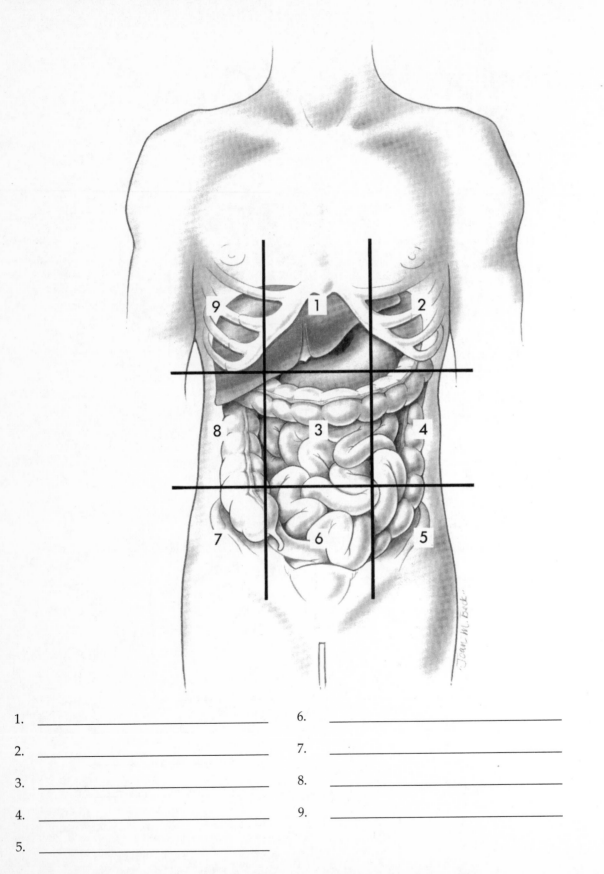

1. _____

2. _____

3. _____

4. _____

5. _____

6. _____

7. _____

8. _____

9. _____

CHAPTER 2

Chemistry of Life

Although anatomy can be studied without knowledge of chemistry, it is hard to imagine an understanding of physiology without a basic comprehension of chemical reactions in the body. Trillions of cells make up the various levels of organization in the body. Our health and survival depends upon the proper chemical maintenance in the cytoplasm of our cells.

Chemists use the terms *elements* or *compounds* to describe all of the substances (matter) in and around us. Distinguishing these two terms is the fact that an element cannot be broken down. A compound, on the other hand, is made up of two or more elements and can be broken down into the elements that form it.

Organic and inorganic compounds are equally important to us. Without organic compounds such as carbohydrates, proteins, and fats, and inorganic compounds such as water, we could not sustain life.

Because we cannot see many of the chemical reactions that take place daily in our bodies, it is sometimes difficult to comprehend the principles involved in initiating them. Chemicals are responsible for directing virtually all of our bodily functions. Therefore, it is important to master the fundamental concepts of chemistry.

TOPICS FOR REVIEW

Before progressing to Chapter 3, you should have an understanding of the basic chemical reactions in the body and the fundamental concepts of biochemistry.

LEVELS OF CHEMICAL ORGANIZATION

Multiple Choice

Circle the correct answer.

1. Which of the following is *not* a subatomic particle?
   A. Proton
   B. Electron
   C. Isotope
   D. Neutron

2. Electrons move about within certain limits called:
   A. Energy levels
   B. Orbitals
   C. Chemical bonding
   D. Shells

3. The number of protons in the nucleus is an atom's:
   A. Atomic mass
   B. Atomic energy level
   C. Atomic number
   D. None of the above

4. The number of protons and neutrons combined is the atom's:
   A. Atomic mass
   B. Atomic energy level
   C. Orbit
   D. Chemical bonding

5. Which of the following is *not* one of the major elements present in the human body?
   A. Oxygen
   B. Carbon
   C. Nitrogen
   D. Iron

6. Atoms usually unite with each other to form larger chemical units called:
   A. Energy levels
   B. Mass
   C. Molecules
   D. Shells

7. Substances whose molecules have more than one element in them are called:
   A. Compounds
   B. Orbitals
   C. Elements
   D. Neutrons

True or False

If the following statement is true, insert "T" in the answer blank. If the statement is false, circle the incorrect word(s) and insert the correct word(s) in the answer blank.

_____ 8. *Matter* is anything that occupies space and has mass.

_____ 9. In the body, most chemicals are in the form of electrons.

_____ 10. At the core of each atom is a nucleus composed of positively charged protons and negatively charged neutrons.

_____ 11. Orbitals are arranged into *energy levels* depending on their distance from the nucleus.

_____ 12. The *formula* for a compound contains symbols for the elements in each molecule.

▶ *If you had difficulty with this section, review pages 21 and 22.*

CHEMICAL BONDING

Multiple Choice

Circle the correct answer.

13. Ionic bonds are chemical bonds formed by the:
    A. Sharing of electrons between atoms
    B. Donation of protons from one atom to another
    C. Donation of electrons from one atom to another
    D. Acceptance of protons from one atom to another

14. Molecules that form ions when dissolved in water are called:
    A. Covalent bonds
    B. Electrolytes
    C. Isotopes
    D. Ionic bonds

15. When atoms share electrons, a/an _____ forms.
    A. Covalent bond
    B. Electrolyte
    C. Ionic bond
    D. Isotope

16. Covalent bonds:
    A. Break apart easily in water
    B. Are not easily broken
    C. Donate electrons
    D. None of the above

17. An example of an ionic bond is:
    A. NaCl
    B. Ca
    C. O
    D. P

18. If a molecule "dissociates" in water, it:
    A. Has taken on additional ions
    B. Has eliminated ions
    C. Separates to form free ions
    D. Forms a covalent bond

▷ *If you had difficulty with this section, review pages 22-25.*

INORGANIC CHEMISTRY

Match each term with its corresponding description or definition.

_____ 19. A type of compound	A. Aqueous solution
_____ 20. Compound most essential to life	B. Water
_____ 21. Dissolves solutes	C. ATP
_____ 22. Water plus common salt	D. Base
_____ 23. Reactants combine only after (H) and (O) atoms removed	E. Solvent
_____ 24. Combine to form a larger product	F. pH
_____ 25. The reverse of dehydration synthesis	G. Dehydration synthesis
_____ 26. Yields energy for muscle contraction	H. Inorganic
_____ 27. Alkaline compound	I. Weak acid
_____ 28. A measure of the H+ concentration	J. Hydrolysis
_____ 29. Easily dissociates to form H+ ions	K. Strong acid
_____ 30. Dissociates very little	L. Reactants

▷ *If you had difficulty with this section, review pages 26-28.*

ORGANIC CHEMISTRY

Circle the correct answer.

A. Carbohydrate   B. Lipid   C. Protein   D. Nucleic acid

_____ 31. Monosaccharide

_____ 32. Triglyceride

_____ 33. DNA

_____ 34. Cholesterol

_____ 35. Amino acid

_____ 36. Glycogen

_____ 37. Sucrose

_____ 38. Phospholipid

_____ 39. Contains C, O, H, and N

_____ 40. RNA

▷ *If you had difficulty with this section, review pages 28-34.*

Fill in the crossword puzzle.

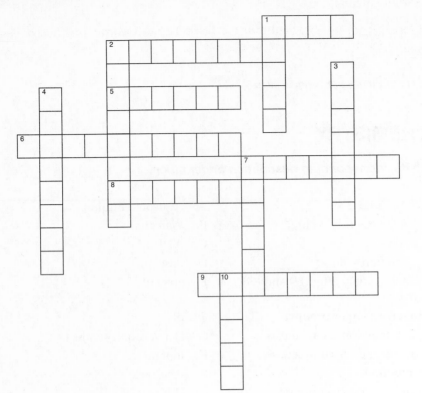

Across
1. Below 7.0 on pH scale
2. Bond formed by sharing electrons
5. Occupies space and has mass
6. Reverse of dehydration synthesis
7. Substances composed of one type of atom
8. Uncharged subatomic particle
9. Subatomic particle

Down
1. Combine to form molecules
2. Substances whose molecules have more than one element
3. Amino acid
4. Polysaccharide
7. Chemical catalyst
10. Fat

APPLYING WHAT YOU KNOW

41. Kim just finished preparing a meal of pan-fried hamburgers for her family. While the frying pan was still hot, she poured the liquid grease into a metal container to cool. Later, she noticed that the liquid oil had solidified as it cooled. Explain the chemistry of why the now room-temperature fat was solid.

42. Carol was gaining weight, yet she was eating very little. Her physician suspected hypothyroidism and suggested a test that measures radiation emitted by the thyroid when radioactive iodine is introduced into the gland. Describe what the radiologist will do to evaluate Carol's thyroid function.

43. Word Find

Can you find the 12 terms from the chapter that are listed below? Words may be spelled top to bottom, bottom to top, right to left, left to right, or diagonally.

Alkaline
Atomic mass
Base
Carbohydrate
Dehydration
Dissociation

Electrolyte
Molecule
Nucleic acid
Proton
Reactant
Solvent

```
E  T  A  R  D  Y  H  O  B  R  A  C  E
T  B  H  S  I  H  L  I  N  A  T  O  D
B  N  E  H  S  G  O  U  L  P  O  T  E
R  Z  A  M  S  F  R  K  U  S  M  T  H
P  R  O  T  O  N  A  I  E  C  I  X  Y
B  R  N  U  C  L  E  I  C  A  C  I  D
C  A  F  T  I  A  E  W  G  G  M  W  R
L  E  S  N  A  B  E  C  E  E  A  E  A
G  Q  E  E  T  E  A  R  U  S  S  F  T
Q  R  P  V  I  B  Y  K  I  L  S  W  I
E  T  Y  L  O  R  T  C  E  L  E  B  O
S  B  U  O  N  E  S  P  N  B  R  B  N
O  P  J  S  T  D  J  M  O  L  U  H  D
```

DID YOU KNOW?

After a vigorous workout, your triglycerides fall 10–20% and your HDL increases by the same percentage for 2-3 hours.

CHECK YOUR KNOWLEDGE

Fill in the blanks.

1. _____ is the field of science devoted to studying the chemical aspects of life.

2. Atoms are composed of protons, electrons, and _____.

3. The farther an orbital extends from the nucleus, the _____ its energy level.

4. Substances can be classified as _____ or _____.

5. Chemical bonds form to make atoms more _____.

6. A(n) _____ is an electrically charged atom.

7. Few _____ compounds have carbon atoms in them and none nave C-C or C-H bonds.

8. _____ is a reaction in which water is lost from the reactants.

9. Chemists often use a _____ to represent a chemical reaction.

10. High levels of _____ in the blood make the blood more acidic.

11. _____ are compounds that produce an excess of H+ ions.

12. _____ maintain pH balance by preventing sudden changes in the H+ ion concentration.

13. _____ literally means "carbon" and "water."

14. _____ is a steroid lipid.

15. Collagen and keratin are examples of _____ proteins.

16. A _____ _____ _____ is formed when the twists and folds of the secondary structure fold again to form a three-dimensional structure.

17. A _____ _____ _____ is a sequence of amino acids in a chain.

CHAPTER 3

Cells and Tissues

ells are the smallest structural units of living things. Therefore, because we are living, we are made up of a mass of cells. Human cells, which vary in shape and size, can only be seen under a microscope. The three main parts of a cell are the cytoplasmic membrane, the cytoplasm, and the nucleus. As you review this chapter, you will be amazed at the resemblance of a cell to the body as a whole. You will identify miniature circulatory systems, reproductive systems, digestive systems, power plants (much like muscular systems), and many other structures that will aid in your understanding of these body systems in future chapters.

Cells—just like humans—require water, food, gases, the elimination of wastes, and numerous other substances and processes in order to survive. The movement of these substances into and out of cells is accomplished by two primary methods: passive transport processes and active transport processes. In passive transport processes, no cellular energy is required to effect movement through the cell membrane. However, in active transport processes, cellular energy is required to provide movement through the cell membrane.

The study of cell reproduction completes this chapter's overview of cells. A basic explanation of DNA, "the hereditary molecule," provides a proper respect for the capability of the cell to transmit physical and mental traits from generation to generation. Reproduction of the cell—mitosis—is a complex process made up of several stages. These stages are outlined and diagrammed in the text to facilitate learning.

This chapter concludes with a discussion of tissues that reviews the four main types of tissues: epithelial, connective, muscle, and nervous. Knowledge of the characteristics, location, and function of these tissues is necessary to complete your understanding of the next structural level of organization.

TOPICS FOR REVIEW

Before progressing to Chapter 4, you should have an understanding of the structure and function of the smallest living unit in the body—the cell. Your review should also include the methods by which substances move through the cell membrane and the stages that occur during cell reproduction. As you finish this chapter, you should have an understanding of tonicity and body tissues and the function they perform in the body.

CELLS

Match the term on the left with the proper selection on the right.

Group A

_____ 1. Cytoplasm

_____ 2. Plasma membrane

_____ 3. Cholesterol

_____ 4. Nucleus

_____ 5. Centrioles

A. Component of plasma membrane

B. Controls reproduction of the cell

C. "Living matter"

D. Paired organelles

E. Surrounds cells

Group B

_____ 6. Ribosomes

_____ 7. Endoplasmic reticulum

_____ 8. Mitochondria

_____ 9. Lysosomes

_____ 10. Golgi apparatus

A. "Power plants"

B. "Digestive bags"

C. "Chemical processing and packaging center"

D. "Protein factories"

E. "Smooth and rough"

Fill in the blanks.

11. The fat molecule _____ helps stabilize the phospholipid molecules to prevent breakage of the plasma membrane.

12. A procedure performed prior to transplanting an organ from one individual to another is _____ _____.

13. Fine, hairlike extensions found on the exposed or free surfaces of some cells are called _____.

14. This organelle is distinguished by the fact that it has two types. It may be either smooth or rough. _____

15. _____ are usually attached to the rough endoplasmic reticulum and produce enzymes and other protein compounds.

16. The _____ provide energy-releasing chemical reactions that go on continuously.

17. The organelles that can digest and destroy microbes that invade the cell are called _____.

18. Mucus is an example of a product manufactured by the _____ _____.

19. These rod-shaped structures, _____, play an important role during cell division.

20. _____ _____ are threadlike structures made up of proteins and DNA.

21. When the immune system mounts a significant attack against the donated tissue, a _____ _____ occurs.

22. The procedure used to test for the presence of antibodies produced in response to the HIV virus is known as _____.

▷ *If you have had difficulty with this section, review pages 41-49 and page 70.*

MOVEMENT OF SUBSTANCES THROUGH CELL MEMBRANES

Circle the correct answer.

23. The energy required for active transport processes is obtained from:
    A. ATP
    B. DNA
    C. Diffusion
    D. Osmosis

24. An example of a passive transport process is:
    A. Permease system
    B. Phagocytosis
    C. Pinocytosis
    D. Diffusion

25. Movement of substances from a region of high concentration to a region of low concentration is known as:
    A. Active transport
    B. Passive transport
    C. Cellular energy
    D. Concentration gradient

26. Osmosis is the _____ of water across a selectively permeable membrane.
    A. Filtration
    B. Equilibrium
    C. Active transport
    D. Diffusion

27. _____ involves the movement of solutes across a selectively permeable membrane by the process of diffusion.
    A. Osmosis
    B. Filtration
    C. Dialysis
    D. Phagocytosis

28. A specialized example of diffusion is:
    A. Osmosis
    B. Permease system
    C. Filtration
    D. All of the above

29. This movement always occurs down a hydrostatic pressure gradient.
    A. Osmosis
    B. Filtration
    C. Dialysis
    D. Facilitated diffusion

30. The uphill movement of a substance through a living cell membrane is:
    A. Osmosis
    B. Diffusion
    C. Active transport process
    D. Passive transport process

31. The ion pump is an example of this type of movement.
    A. Gravity
    B. Hydrostatic pressure
    C. Active transport process
    D. Passive transport process

32. An example of a cell that uses phagocytosis is the:
    A. White blood cell
    B. Red blood cell
    C. Muscle cell
    D. Bone cell

33. A salt solution that contains a higher concentration of salt than living red blood cells would be:
    A. Hypotonic
    B. Hypertonic
    C. Isotonic
    D. Homeostatic

34. A red blood cell becomes engorged with water and will eventually lyse, releasing hemoglobin into the solution. This solution is _____ to the red blood cell.
    A. Hypotonic
    B. Hypertonic
    C. Isotonic
    D. Homeostatic

▷ *If you have had difficulty with this section, review pages 49-55.*

CELL REPRODUCTION AND HEREDITY

Circle the one that does not belong.

35. DNA	Adenine	Uracil	Thymine
36. Complementary base pairing	Guanine	RNA	Cytosine
37. Anaphase	Specific sequence	Gene	Base pairs
38. RNA	Ribose	Thymine	Uracil
39. Translation	Protein synthesis	mRNA	Interphase
40. Cleavage furrow	Anaphase	Prophase	2 daughter cells
41. "Resting"	Prophase	Interphase	DNA replication
42. Identical	2 nuclei	Telophase	Metaphase
43. Metaphase	Prophase	Telophase	Gene

▶ *If you have had difficulty with this section, review pages 55-62.*

TISSUES

44. Fill in the missing areas of the chart.

TISSUE	LOCATION	FUNCTION
Epithelial		
1. Simple squamous	1a. Alveoli of lungs	1a.
	1b. Lining of blood and lymphatic vessels	1b.
2. Stratified squamous	2a.	2a. Protection
	2b.	2b. Protection
3. Simple columnar	3.	3. Protection, secretion, absorption
4.	4. Urinary bladder	4. Protection
5. Pseudostratified	5.	5. Protection
6. Simple cuboidal	6. Glands; kidney tubules	6.

Connective		
1. Areolar	1.	1. Connection
2.	2. Under skin	2. Protection; insulation
3. Dense fibrous	3. Tendons; ligaments; fascia; scar tissue	3.
4. Bone	4.	4. Support, protection
5. Cartilage	5.	5. Firm but flexible support
6. Blood	6. Blood vessels	6.
7.	7. Red bone marrow	7. Blood cell formation
Muscle		
1. Skeletal (striated voluntary)	1.	1. Movement of bones
2.	2. Wall of heart	2. Contraction of heart
3. Smooth	3.	3. Movement of substances along ducts; change in diameter of pupils and shape of lens; "gooseflesh"
Nervous		
1.	1.	1. Irritability, conduction

▷ *If you have had difficulty with this section, review Tables 3-7, 3-8, and 3-9 and pages 62-74.*

APPLYING WHAT YOU KNOW

45. Mr. Fee's boat had capsized, and he was stranded on a deserted shoreline for 2 days without food or water. When found, he had swallowed a great deal of seawater. He was taken to the emergency room in a state of dehydration. In the space below, draw the appearance of Mr. Fee's red blood cells as they would appear to the laboratory technician.

46. The nurse was instructed to dissolve a pill in a small amount of liquid medication. As she dropped the capsule into the liquid, she was interrupted by the telephone. On her return to the medication cart, she found the medication completely dissolved and apparently scattered evenly throughout the liquid. This phenomenon did not surprise her since she was aware from her knowledge of cell transport that _____ had created this distribution.

47. Ms. Bence has emphysema and has been admitted to the hospital unit with oxygen per nasal cannula. Emphysema destroys the tiny air sacs in the lungs. These tiny air sacs, alveoli, provide what function for Ms. Bence?

48. Merrily was 5'4" and weighed 115 lbs. She appeared very healthy and fit, yet her doctor advised her that she was "overfat." What might be the explanation for this assessment?

49.   Word Find

Can you find the 16 terms from this chapter that are listed below? Words may be spelled top to bottom, bottom to top, right to left, left to right, or diagonally.

```
A  P  D  I  E  V  E  W  N  P  F  E  H  Y  X
I  G  I  Z  N  S  R  L  X  S  T  W  F  Z  S
R  J  V  N  N  T  A  I  L  M  R  P  H  M  F
D  W  U  E  O  O  E  H  B  E  A  D  U  G  F
N  W  I  U  I  C  I  R  P  O  N  N  F  B  W
O  P  U  R  S  H  Y  T  P  O  S  A  W  X  K
H  X  F  O  U  R  Y  T  A  H  L  O  G  A  W
C  L  Z  N  F  O  Y  P  O  R  A  E  M  R  M
O  U  I  X  F  M  L  F  O  S  T  S  T  E  O
T  T  B  Y  I  A  B  C  O  T  I  L  E  S  D
I  V  S  O  D  T  T  M  I  T  O  S  I  S  U
M  N  A  A  I  I  L  E  N  L  N  N  F  R
E  O  K  K  I  D  C  Q  H  B  I  V  I  T  H
E  K  T  X  B  Z  A  E  A  L  S  A  E  C  K
S  B  Z  R  P  M  V  L  X  W  Z  A  Z  C  V
```

Chromatid	Hypotonic	Pinocytosis
Cilia	Interphase	Ribosome
Cuboidal	Mitochondria	Telophase
DNA	Mitosis	Translation
Diffusion	Neuron	
Filtration	Organelle	

DID YOU KNOW?

The largest single cell in the human body is the female sex cell, the ovum. The smallest single cell in the human body is the male sex cell, the sperm.

CELLS AND TISSUES

Fill in the crossword puzzle.

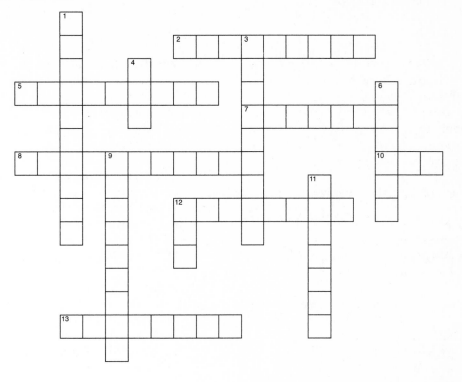

Across

2. Last stage of mitosis
5. Shriveling of cell due to water withdrawal
7. Fat
8. Cartilage cell
10. Ribonucleic acid (abbreviation)
12. Specialized example of diffusion
13. First stage of mitosis

Down

1. Having an osmotic pressure greater than that of the solution with which it is compared
3. Cell organ
4. Energy source for active transport
6. Nerve cell
9. Occurs when substances scatter themselves evenly throughout an available space
11. Reproduction process of most cells
12. Chemical "blueprint" of the body (abbreviation)

CHECK YOUR KNOWLEDGE

Multiple Choice

Circle the correct answer.

1. Which of the following cellular structures has the ability to secrete digestive enzymes?
   A. Lysosomes
   B. Mitochondria
   C. Golgi apparatus
   D. Ribosomes

2. Red blood cells do what when placed in a hypertonic salt solution?
   A. Remain unchanged
   B. Undergo crenation
   C. Lyse
   D. None of the above

3. Which of the following statements is true of chromatin granules?
    A. They exist in the cell cytoplasm.
    B. They are made up of DNA.
    C. They form spindle fibers.
    D. All of the above

4. In which stage of mitosis do chromosomes move to opposite ends of the cell along the spindle fibers?
    A. Anaphase
    B. Metaphase
    C. Prophase
    D. Telophase

5. Filtration is a process that involves which of the following?
    A. Active transport
    B. The expenditure of energy
    C. Changes in hydrostatic pressure
    D. All of the above

6. The synthesis of proteins by ribosomes using information coded in the mRNA molecule is called what?
    A. Translation
    B. Transcription
    C. Replication
    D. Crenation

7. Which of the following is *not* an example of connective tissue?
    A. Muscle
    B. Blood
    C. Fat
    D. Bone

8. Which of the following is the most abundant and widely distributed type of body tissue?
    A. Epithelial
    B. Connective
    C. Muscle
    D. Nerve

9. Simple, squamous epithelial tissue is made up of which of the following?
    A. A single layer of long, narrow cells
    B. Several layers of long, narrow cells
    C. A single layer of flat, scale-like cells
    D. Several layers of flat, scale-like cells

10. Which of the following groupings is correct when describing one of the muscle cell types?
    A. Visceral, striated, involuntary
    B. Skeletal, smooth, voluntary
    C. Cardiac, smooth, involuntary
    D. Skeletal, striated, voluntary

Matching

Select the most appropriate answer in column B for each item in column A. (Only one answer is correct.)

Column A

_____ 11. Haversian system
_____ 12. Plasma membrane
_____ 13. Neuron
_____ 14. Pinocytosis
_____ 15. Prophase
_____ 16. Adenine
_____ 17. Diffusion
_____ 18. Squamous
_____ 19. Mitochondria
_____ 20. Tendon

Column B

A. Chromatids
B. Thymine
C. Active transport
D. Energy
E. Fibrous
F. Bone
G. Phospholipids
H. Flat
I. Passive transport
J. Axon

CELL STRUCTURE

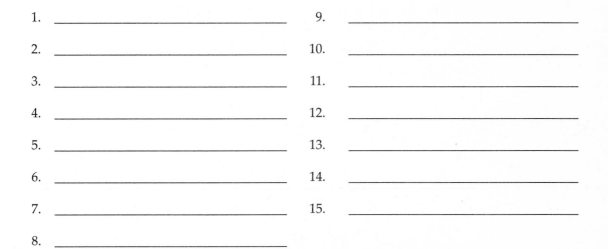

1. _____
2. _____
3. _____
4. _____
5. _____
6. _____
7. _____
8. _____

9. _____
10. _____
11. _____
12. _____
13. _____
14. _____
15. _____

MITOSIS

1. _____   4. _____

2. _____   5. _____

3. _____   6. _____

TISSUES

1. _____

2. _____

3. _____

4. _____

5. _____

6. _____

7. _____

8. _____

9. _____

10. _____

11. _____

12. _____

Organ Systems of the Body

A smooth-running automobile is the result of many systems working together harmoniously. The engine, the fuel system, the exhaust system, the brake system, and the cooling system are but a few of the many complex structural units that the automobile as a whole relies on to keep it functioning smoothly. So it is with the human body. We, too, depend on the successful performance of many individual systems working together to create and maintain a healthy human being.

When you have completed your review of the 11 major organ systems and the organs that make up these systems, you will find your understanding of the performance of the body as a whole much more meaningful.

TOPICS FOR REVIEW

Before progressing to Chapter 5, you should have an understanding of the 11 major organ systems and be able to identify the organs that are included in each system. Your review should also include current approaches to organ replacement.

ORGAN SYSTEMS OF THE BODY

Match the term on the left with the proper selection on the right.

Group A

_____ 1.	Integumentary	A. Hair
_____ 2.	Skeletal	B. Spinal cord
_____ 3.	Muscular	C. Hormones
_____ 4.	Nervous	D. Tendons
_____ 5.	Endocrine	E. Joints

Group B

_____ 6.	Cardiovascular	A. Esophagus
_____ 7.	Lymphatic	B. Ureters
_____ 8.	Urinary	C. Larynx
_____ 9.	Digestive	D. Genitalia
_____ 10.	Respiratory	E. Spleen
_____ 11.	Reproductive	F. Capillaries

Circle the one that does not belong.

12.	Pharynx	Trachea	Mouth	Alveoli
13.	Uterus	Rectum	Gonads	Prostate
14.	Veins	Arteries	Heart	Pancreas
15.	Pineal	Bladder	Ureters	Urethra
16.	Tendon	Smooth	Joints	Voluntary
17.	Pituitary	Brain	Spinal cord	Nerves
18.	Cartilage	Joints	Ligaments	Tendons
19.	Hormones	Pituitary	Pancreas	Appendix
20.	Thymus	Nails	Hair	Oil glands
21.	Esophagus	Pharynx	Mouth	Trachea
22.	Thymus	Spleen	Tonsils	Liver

Fill in the missing areas.

SYSTEM	ORGANS	FUNCTIONS
23. Integumentary	Skin, nails, hair, sense receptors, sweat glands, oil glands	
24. Skeletal		Support, movement, storage of minerals, blood formation
25. Muscular	Muscles	
26.	Brain, spinal cord, nerves	Communication, integration, control, recognition of sensory stimuli
27. Endocrine		Secretion of hormones; communication, integration, control
28. Cardiovascular	Heart, blood vessels	
29. Lymphatic		Transportation, immune system
30.	Kidneys, ureters, bladder, urethra	Elimination of wastes, electrolyte balance, acid-base balance, water balance
31. Digestive		Digestion of food, absorption of nutrients
32.	Nose, pharynx, larynx, trachea, bronchi, lungs	Exchange of gases in the lungs
33. Reproductive		Survival of species; production of sex cells, fertilization, development, birth; nourishment of offspring; production of hormones

 If you have had difficulty with this section, review pages 85-101 and the chapter summary on pages 105-107.

ORGAN TRANSPLANTATION

Fill in the blanks.

34. An organ not required for life to continue is a _____

_____.

35. Many people suffering from deafness have had their hearing partially restored by "artificial ears" called

_____ _____.

36. One of the earliest devices to augment vital functions was the "artificial kidney" or

_____ _____.

37. Electromechanical devices that help keep blood pumping in patients suffering from end-stage heart disease are known as _____.

38. One approach that offers the hope of a permanent solution to loss of vital organ function is

_____ _____.

39. After cancerous breasts are removed, "new" breasts can be formed from skin and muscle tissue using a method known as _____ _____.

40. The advantage to using a patient's own tissues in organ replacement is that the possibility of

_____ is eliminated.

▶ *If you have had difficulty with this section, review pages 101-104.*

UNSCRAMBLE THE WORDS

41. **R T A H E**

42. **I E P L N A**

43. **E E N V R**

44. **S U H E S O P G A**

Take the circled letters, unscramble them, and fill in the statement.

The more thoroughly you review this chapter, the less

45. ☐☐☐☐☐☐☐ **you will be during your test.**

APPLYING WHAT YOU KNOW

46. Myrna was 15 years old and had not yet started menstruating. Her family physician decided to consult two other physicians, each of whom specialized in a different system. Specialists in the areas of _____ and _____ were consulted.

47. Brian was admitted to the hospital with second- and third-degree burns over 50% of his body. He was placed in isolation. When Jenny went to visit him, she was required to wear a hospital gown and mask. Why was Brian placed in isolation? Why was Jenny required to wear special attire?

48. Sheila had a mastectomy to remove a cancerous lesion in her breast. Her body rejected the breast implant used to reconstruct her breast. Is there another breast reconstruction option to offer Sheila? If so, explain this option.

49.   Word Find

Can you find the 11 organ systems? Words may be spelled top to bottom, bottom to top, right to left, left to right, or diagonally.

```
Y  R  A  T  N  E  M  U  G  E  T  N  I  R  F
H  N  E  R  V  O  U  S  K  I  R  J  M  G  T
L  Y  M  P  H  A  T  I  C  I  S  Y  Y  U  I
B  N  X  Y  R  O  T  A  L  U  C  R  I  C  W
P  E  L  R  E  O  M  J  M  S  O  M  M  P  S
C  C  W  M  A  N  D  L  A  T  E  L  E  K  S
R  R  K  E  M  L  I  U  A  A  V  V  U  K  N
D  K  X  P  D  J  U  R  C  J  I  R  Q  E  M
C  D  B  V  C  V  I  C  C  T  T  K  W  C  X
X  R  Q  Q  D  P  H  C  S  O  I  X  P  A  Z
M  F  M  U  S  Y  D  E  V  U  D  V  Y  K  E
U  E  S  E  C  Z  G  T  Q  D  M  N  E  K  O
P  Y  R  A  N  I  R  U  C  T  C  N  E  W  H
N  H  T  N  D  E  P  S  I  X  A  Q  O  I  E
```

Circulatory	Lymphatic	Respiratory
Digestive	Muscular	Skeletal
Endocrine	Nervous	Urinary
Integumentary	Reproductive	

DID YOU KNOW?

Muscles comprise 40% of your body weight. Your skeleton, however, only accounts for 18% of your body weight.

ORGAN SYSTEMS

Fill in the crossword puzzle.

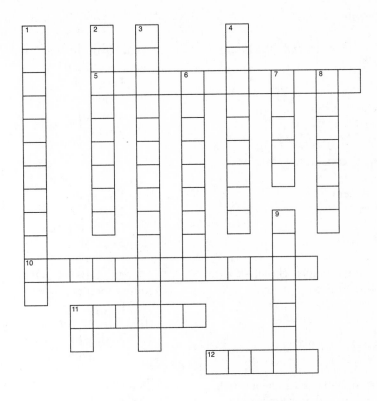

ACROSS

5. Specialized signal of nervous system (two words)
10. Skin
11. Testes and ovaries
12. Undigested residue of digestion

DOWN

1. Inflammation of the appendix
2. Vulva, penis, and scrotum
3. Heart and blood vessels
4. Subdivision of circulatory system
6. System of hormones
7. Waste product of kidneys
8. Agent that causes change in the activity of a structure
9. Chemical secretion of endocrine system
11. Gastrointestinal tract (abbreviation)

CHECK YOUR KNOWLEDGE

Multiple Choice

Circle the correct answer.

1. Which body system serves to clean the blood of waste products?
   A. Digestive
   B. Endocrine
   C. Cardiovascular
   D. Urinary

2. Ovaries and testes are considered components of which system?
   A. Reproductive system
   B. Endocrine system
   C. Both A and B
   D. None of the above

3. Which of the following organs is classified as an accessory organ of the digestive system?
   A. Mouth
   B. Esophagus
   C. Tongue
   D. Anal canal

4. Factors in the environment such as heat, light, pressure, and temperature that can be recognized by the nervous system are called:
   A. Effectors
   B. Stimuli
   C. Receptors
   D. Nerve impulses

5. Which body system stores the mineral calcium?
   A. Cardiovascular
   B. Digestive
   C. Lymphatic
   D. Skeletal

6. What is undigested material in the gastrointestinal tract called?
   A. Feces
   B. Urine
   C. Lymph
   D. Blood

7. Which body system produces heat and maintains body posture?
   A. Endocrine
   B. Muscular
   C. Cardiovascular
   D. Skeletal

8. Which of the following is *not* a function of the integumentary system?
   A. Integration
   B. Temperature regulation
   C. Ability to serve as a sense organ
   D. Protection

9. Which of the following is *not* a component of the digestive system?
   A. Spleen
   B. Liver
   C. Pancreas
   D. Gallbladder

10. When a group of tissues starts working together to perform a common function, what level of organization is achieved?
    A. Systemic
    B. Tissue
    C. Organ
    D. Cellular

Matching

Select the most appropriate answer in column B for each item in column A. (There is only one correct answer.)

Column A

_____ 11. Sweat glands

_____ 12. Heart

_____ 13. Spleen

_____ 14. Vas deferens

_____ 15. Bladder

_____ 16. Gallbladder

_____ 17. Uterine tubes

_____ 18. Trachea

_____ 19. Spinal cord

_____ 20. Adrenals

Column B

A. Endocrine

B. Urinary

C. Integumentary

D. Cardiovascular

E. Respiratory

F. Digestive

G. Male reproductive

H. Lymphatic

I. Female reproductive

J. Nervous

CHAPTER 5

Mechanisms of Disease

O ne of our foremost concerns is health. We are fascinated and constantly confronted with information regarding what is necessary to be in good health, what is required for proper maintenance of the body, and what behaviors are responsible for disease.

Organisms play an important role in health. They are microscopic structures that are present everywhere. We need some organisms in the preparation of foods, in industry and agriculture, in connection with the problems of shelter or clothing, and in combating disease. However, many organisms are responsible for disease. They attack and disturb the normal homeostasis of the body and adversely affect our health. Many varieties of organisms exist. They are often classified by shape, size, function, or staining properties. To prevent disease, we must prevent pathogenic or disease-producing organisms from entering the body. This is not an easy task because we are surrounded by pathogenic organisms. It is important that we understand the transmission and control of these organisms to fully comprehend the mechanisms of disease.

TOPICS FOR REVIEW

Before progressing to Chapter 6 you should familiarize yourself with disease terminology and patterns of disease. You should continue your review by studying pathophysiology and pathogenic organisms. Finally, an understanding of tumors, cancer, and inflammation is necessary to conclude your knowledge of this chapter.

STUDYING DISEASE

Match the term on the left with the proper selection on the right.

Group A

_____ 1. Pathology   A. Subjective abnormalities
_____ 2. Signs   B. Study of disease
_____ 3. Symptoms   C. Collection of different signs and symptoms that present a clear picture of a pathological condition
_____ 4. Syndrome   D. Study of factors involved in causing a disease
_____ 5. Etiology   E. Objective abnormalities

Group B

_____ 6. Latent   A. Recovery
_____ 7. Convalescence   B. Disease native to a local region
_____ 8. Pandemics   C. "Hidden" stage
_____ 9. Endemic   D. Affects large geographic regions
_____ 10. Pathogenesis   E. Actual pattern of a disease's development

▶ *If you have had difficulty with this section, review pages 111-113.*

PATHOPHYSIOLOGY

Fill in the blanks.

11. _____ is the organized study of the underlying physiological processes associated with disease.

12. Many diseases are best understood as disturbances of _____.

13. Altered or _____ genes can cause abnormal proteins to be made.

14. An organism that lives in or on another organism to obtain its nutrients is called a _____.

15. Abnormal tissue growths may also be referred to as _____.

16. *Autoimmunity* literally means _____.

17. Genetic factors, age, lifestyle, stress, environmental factors, and preexisting conditions are _____ _____ that may be responsible for predisposing a person to disease.

18. Scientists at the _____ _____ _____ _____ continuously track the incidence and spread of disease in this country and worldwide.

19. Conditions caused by psychological factors are sometimes called _____ disorders.

20. A primary condition can put a person at risk for developing a _____ condition.

▶ *If you have difficulty with this section, review pages 113-116.*

PATHOGENIC ORGANISMS

Circle the correct answer.

21. The smallest of all pathogens—microscopic nonliving particles—are called:
    A. Bacteria
    B. Fungi
    C. Viruses
    D. Protozoa

22. A tiny, primitive cell without a nucleus is called a:
    A. Bacterium
    B. Fungus
    C. Virus
    D. Protozoa

23. An example of a viral disease is:
    A. Diarrhea
    B. Mononucleosis
    C. Syphilis
    D. Toxic shock syndrome

24. Bacteria that require oxygen for metabolism are classified as:
    A. Gram positive
    B. Gram negative
    C. Aerobic
    D. Anaerobic

25. Bacilli are shaped like:
    A. Spheres
    B. Curves
    C. Squares
    D. Rods

26. Without chlorophyll, _____ cannot produce their own food, so they must consume or parasitize other organisms.
    A. Bacteria
    B. Fungi
    C. Viruses
    D. Protozoa

27. Protozoa include:
    A. Amoebas
    B. Flagellates
    C. Ciliates
    D. All of the above

28. Pathogenic animals include the following:
    A. Nematodes
    B. Platyhelminths
    C. Arthropods
    D. All of the above

29. The key to preventing diseases caused by pathogenic organisms is to:
    A. Have an annual physical
    B. Stop them from entering the body
    C. Isolate yourself from all disease-carrying individuals
    D. None of the above

30. The destruction of all living organisms is known as:
    A. Disinfection
    B. Antisepsis
    C. Sterilization
    D. Isolation

31. Ways in which pathogens can spread include:
    A. Person-to-person contact
    B. Environmental contact
    C. Opportunistic invasion
    D. Transmission by vector
    E. All of the above

32. Compounds produced by certain living organisms that kill or inhibit pathogens are:
    A. Antiseptics
    B. Antibiotics
    C. Disinfectants
    D. Sterilizers

▶ *If you have had difficulty with this section, review pages 116-126.*

TUMORS AND CANCER

Circle the correct answer.

33. Benign tumors usually grow (slowly or quickly).

34. Malignant tumors (are or are not) encapsulated.

35. An example of a benign tumor that arises from epithelial tissue is (papilloma or lipoma).

36. A general term for malignant tumors that arise from connective tissues is (melanoma or sarcoma).

37. Abnormal, undifferentiated tumor cells are often produced by a process called (hyperplasia or anaplasia).

38. A cancer specialist is an (osteologist or oncologist).

39. The Papanicolaou test is a (biopsy or MRI).

40. (Staging or Grading) involves classifying a tumor based on its size and the extent of its spread.

41. Cachexia involves a loss of (appetite or hair).

▶ *If you have had difficulty with this section, review pages 126-134.*

WARNING SIGNS OF CANCER

List the eight warning signs of cancer.

42. _____   46. _____
43. _____   47. _____
44. _____   48. _____
45. _____   49. _____

▶ *If you have had difficulty with this section, review page 130.*

INFLAMMATION

If the statement is true, write "T" in the answer blank. If the statement is false, correct the statement by circling the incorrect term and inserting the correct term in the answer blank.

_____ 50. As tissue cells are damaged, they release inflammation mediators such as histamines, prostaglandins, and kinins.

_____ 51. Inflammatory exudate is quickly removed by lymphatic vessels and carried to lymph nodes, which act as filters.

_____ 52. Inflammation mediators can also act as signals that attract red blood cells to the injury site.

_____ 53. The movement of white blood cells in response to chemical attractants is called *chemotaxis*.

_____ 54. When new cells are similar to those that they replace, the process is known as *replacement*.

_____ 55. Fevers usually subside after the irritant has been eliminated.

_____ 56. The fever response in children and in the elderly often differs from that in the normal adult.

▶ *If you have had difficulty with this section, review pages 134-138.*

UNSCRAMBLE THE WORDS

57. **N G F U I**

58. **C E O N O G N E**

59. **A D E E M**

60. **R S P O E**

Take the circled letters, unscramble them, and fill in the statement.

What Mr. Lynch found to be most difficult as a teacher.

61.

APPLYING WHAT YOU KNOW

62. Trent was examined by his doctor and was diagnosed as having a rhinovirus. Does he have need for concern? Why or why not?

63. Julius was 2 years old and was experiencing rectal itching and insomnia. The pediatrician told Julius' mother that he suspected a nematode. What is the common term for the specific nematode that might cause these symptoms?

64. Shirley was cleaning her house and wanted to use the most appropriate and effective aseptic method to prevent the spread of germs. What would you suggest?

65. Mr. and Mrs. Gibbs adopted a child of Chinese descent. Mrs. Gibbs researched the "gene pool" of the child to alert her to any special concerns. What is a "gene pool" and how will this information assist Mr. and Mrs. Gibbs in the rearing of their child?

66. Bill decided to become a paramedic. His application for school suggested that he receive the series of vaccinations for hepatitis B. Why?

67. Word Find

Can you find the 18 terms from this chapter that are listed below? Words may be spelled top to bottom, bottom to top, right to left, left to right, or diagonally.

```
N  P  E  S  D  B  S  L  A  A  C  E  R
W  O  L  S  I  C  I  M  E  D  I  P  E
X  V  I  O  F  S  X  V  R  E  N  A  T
O  D  P  T  U  E  A  D  O  N  C  R  U
H  S  O  V  A  S  T  T  P  O  U  A  C
Y  S  M  P  U  M  O  A  S  M  B  S  A
Y  P  A  R  O  I  M  B  I  A  A  I  I
N  L  I  O  S  R  E  A  F  L  T  T  D
W  V  J  T  C  Z  H  C  L  L  I  E  Y
W  Q  K  O  W  G  C  T  Q  F  O  C  M
V  Q  F  Z  I  F  G  E  R  P  N  F  A
K  E  N  O  Q  E  J  R  B  A  F  I  L
B  B  J  A  F  E  N  I  C  C  A  V  H
W  Z  F  H  R  B  S  U  D  M  Q  D  C
M  X  E  C  K  M  B  M  K  U  O  Z  P
```

Acute	Chlamydia	Metastasis
Adenoma	Ciliate	Parasite
Arthropod	Epidemic	Protozoa
Bacterium	Incubation	Spore
Biopsy	Inflammation	Vaccine
Chemotaxis	Lipoma	Virus

DID YOU KNOW?

As many as 500,000 Americans die from cancer each year, making it the second-leading cause of death after cardiovascular disease. Half of all cancers are diagnosed in people under the age of 67.

The hepatitis B virus (HBV) has infected more than 250 million people worldwide.

MECHANISMS OF DISEASE

Fill in the crossword puzzle.

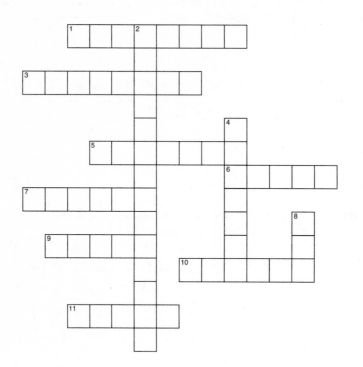

ACROSS

1. Roundworm
3. "Cancer gene"
5. Rod-shaped cells
6. Round cells
7. Spreads disease to other organisms
9. Lack chlorophyll
10. Possess pseudopodia
11. Tissue swelling

DOWN

2. Glandular cancer
4. Microscopic organism
8. Thick inflammatory exudate

CHECK YOUR KNOWLEDGE

Multiple Choice

Circle the correct answer.

1. Diseases with undetermined causes are:
   A. Asymptomatic
   B. Idiopathic
   C. Psychogenic
   D. Predisposing

2. The study of the occurrence, distribution, and transmission of diseases is:
   A. Entomology
   B. Pathology
   C. Oncology
   D. Epidemiology

3. Streptomycin is an example of a/an:
   A. Antibiotic
   B. Vaccine
   C. Pathogenic organism
   D. All of the above

4. Reversal of a chronic condition is called:
   A. Inflammatory response
   B. Predisposing condition
   C. Hemostasis
   D. Remission

5. If antibodies are found in an immunological test, it is assumed that:
   A. The patient has been exposed to a pathogen
   B. The infection is gone
   C. A and B
   D. None of the above

6. An epidemiologist:
   A. Studies the transmission of disease
   B. Monitors infection control programs
   C. Tracks the spread of disease
   D. All of the above

7. Study of the underlying physiological processes associated with disease leads to:
   A. Strategies of prevention
   B. Strategies of treatment
   C. A and B
   D. None of the above

8. Severe loss of appetite, weight loss, and general weakness in a cancer patient describe:
   A. Secondary infection
   B. Cachexia
   C. Inflammatory response
   D. Chemotaxis

9. Intracellular parasites that are not technically living organisms are characteristics of:
   A. Bacteria
   B. Fungi
   C. Amoebas
   D. Viruses

10. Examples of protozoa include all of the following *except*:
    A. Bacilli
    B. Flagellates
    C. Sporozoa
    D. Amoebas

Matching

Select the most appropriate answer in column B for each item in column A. (Only one answer is correct.)

Column A

_____ 11. Syndrome

_____ 12. Metastasis

_____ 13. Anaerobic

_____ 14. Protozoa

_____ 15. Pathogenesis

_____ 16. Fever

_____ 17. Metazoa

_____ 18. Pathology

_____ 19. Neoplasm

_____ 20. Arthropods

Column B

A. Study of disease

B. Require absence of oxygen

C. Collection of signs and symptoms

D. Spread of cancer cells

E. Multicellular organisms that parasitize humans

F. Abnormal cell growth

G. Pattern of disease development

H. Mites

I. Inflammatory response

J. One-celled organisms that parasitize cells

MAJOR GROUPS OF PATHOGENIC BACTERIA

1.

2.

3.

4.

MAJOR GROUPS OF PATHOGENIC PROTOZOA

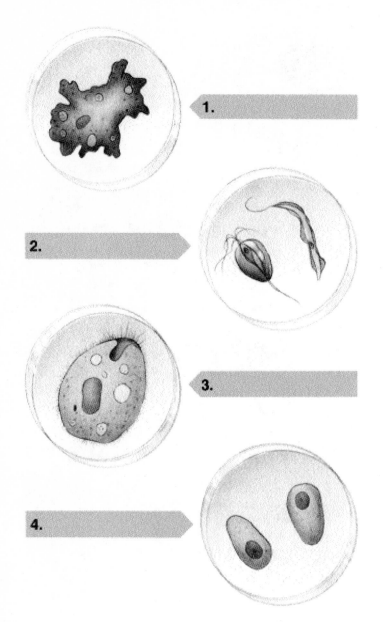

EXAMPLES OF PATHOGENIC ANIMALS

MAJOR GROUPS OF PATHOGENIC FUNGI

1.

2.

CHAPTER 6

The Integumentary System and Body Membranes

More of our time, attention, and money are spent on this system than any other. Every time we look into a mirror we become aware of the integumentary system, as we observe our skin, hair, nails, and the appendages that give luster and comfort to this system. The discussion of the skin begins with the structure and function of the two primary layers called the *epidermis* and *dermis*. It continues with an examination of the appendages of the skin, which include the hair, receptors, nails, sebaceous glands, and sudoriferous glands. Your study of skin concludes with a review of one of the most serious and frequent threats to the skin—burns. An understanding of the integumentary system provides you with an appreciation of the danger that severe burns could pose to this system.

Membranes are thin, sheetlike structures that cover, protect, anchor, or lubricate body surfaces, cavities, or organs. The two major categories of membranes are epithelial and connective. Each type is located in specific areas of the body and each is vulnerable to specific disease conditions. Knowledge of the location and function of these membranes prepares you for the study of their relationship to other systems and the body as a whole.

TOPICS FOR REVIEW

Before progressing to Chapter 7, you should have an understanding of the skin, its appendages, major skin disorders, and infections. Your review should include the classification of burns and the method used to estimate the percentage of body surface area affected by burns. A knowledge of the types of body membranes, their location, and their function is necessary to complete your study of this chapter.

CLASSIFICATION OF BODY MEMBRANES

Select the best answer.

A. Cutaneous   B. Serous   C. Mucous   D. Synovial

_____ 1. Pleura

_____ 2. Lines joint spaces

_____ 3. Respiratory tract

_____ 4. Skin

_____ 5. Peritoneum

_____ 6. Contains no epithelium

_____ 7. Urinary tract

_____ 8. Lines body surfaces that open directly to the exterior

▷ *If you have had difficulty with this section, review pages 147-150.*

THE SKIN

Match the term on the left with the proper selection on the right.

Group A

_____ 9.   Integumentary system
_____ 10. Epidermis
_____ 11. Dermis
_____ 12. Subcutaneous
_____ 13. Cutaneous membrane

A. Outermost layer of skin
B. Deeper of the two layers of skin
C. Hypodermis
D. The skin is the primary organ
E. Composed of dermis and epidermis

Group B

_____ 14. Keratin
_____ 15. Melanin
_____ 16. Stratum corneum
_____ 17. Dermal papillae
_____ 18. Cyanosis

A. Protective protein
B. Blue-gray color of skin resulting from a decrease in oxygen
C. Rows of peglike projections
D. Brown pigment
E. Outer layer of epidermis

Select the best answer.

A. Epidermis   B. Dermis

_____ 19. Tightly packed epithelial cells

_____ 20. Nerves

_____ 21. Fingerprints

_____ 22. Blisters

_____ 23. Keratin

_____ 24. Connective tissue

_____ 25. Follicle

_____ 26. Sebaceous gland

_____ 27. Sweat gland

_____ 28. More cellular than other layer

▶ *If you have had difficulty with this section, review pages 150-163.*

Fill in the blanks.

29. The three most important functions of the skin are _____,
_____, and _____.

30. _____ prevents the sun's ultraviolet rays from penetrating the interior
of the body.

31. The hair of a newborn infant is called _____.

32. Hair growth begins from a small, cap-shaped cluster of cells called the
_____ _____.

33. Hair loss of any kind is called _____.

34. The _____ _____ muscle produces
"goose pimples."

35. A birthmark that appears as a bruise at birth and grows rapidly into a bright red nodule is called a

_____ _____ .

36. The most numerous, important, and widespread sweat glands in the body are the

_____ sweat glands.

37. The _____ sweat glands are found primarily in the axilla and in the pigmented skin areas around the genitals.

38. _____ has been described as "nature's skin cream."

▷ *If you have had difficulty with this section, review pages 150-163.*

Circle the correct answer.

39. A first-degree burn (will or will not) blister.

40. A second-degree burn (will or will not) scar.

41. A third-degree burn (will or will not) have pain immediately.

42. According to the "rule of nines" the body is divided into (9 or 11) areas of 9%.

43. Destruction of the subcutaneous layer occurs in (second- or third-) degree burns.

▷ *If you have had difficulty with this section, review pages 165-167.*

DISORDERS OF THE SKIN

Circle the correct answer.

44. Any disorder of the skin may be called:
    A. Dermatitis
    B. Dermatosis
    C. Dermatotomy
    D. None of the above

45. Any measurable variation from the normal structure of a tissue is known as a/an:
    A. Lesion
    B. Burn
    C. Blister
    D. Erythema

46. An example of a papule is a:
    A. Scratch
    B. Bedsore
    C. Freckle
    D. Wart

47. An example of a skin disorder that may produce fissures is:
    A. Acne
    B. A bedsore
    C. Psoriasis
    D. Athlete's foot

48. The skin is the _____ line of defense against microbes that invade the body's internal environment.
    A. First
    B. Second
    C. Third
    D. Fourth

49. Tinea is a fungal infection and may appear as:
    A. Ringworm
    B. Jock itch
    C. Athlete's foot
    D. All of the above

50. Furuncles are local staphylococci infections and are also known as:
    A. Scabies
    B. Warts
    C. Boils
    D. Impetigo

51. The most common type of skin cancer is:
    A. Squamous cell
    B. Basal cell
    C. Melanoma
    D. Kaposi's sarcoma

▷ *If you had difficulty with this section, review pages 164-172.*

UNSCRAMBLE THE WORDS

52. **P I D E E M I R S**

53. **R E K T A I N**

54. **A H I R**

55. **U G O N A L**

55. **D R T O N I D E H Y A**

Take the circled letters, unscramble
them, and fill in the statement.

What Amanda's mother gave her after every date.

56.

APPLYING WHAT YOU KNOW

58. Mr. Ziven was admitted to the hospital with second- and third-degree burns. Both arms, the anterior trunk, the right anterior leg, and the genital region were affected by the burns. The doctor quickly estimated that _____% of Mr. Ziven's body had been burned.

59. Mrs. James complained to her doctor that she had severe pain in her chest and feared that she was having a heart attack. An ECG revealed nothing unusual, but Mrs. James insisted that every time she took a breath she experienced pain. What might be the cause of Mrs. James' pain?

60. Mrs. Collins was born with a rare condition known as xeroderma pigmentosum. What activity should she avoid?

61. After investigating the scene of the crime, Officer Gorski announced that dermal papillae were found that would help solve the case. What did he mean?

62. Word Find

Can you find the 15 terms from this chapter that are listed below? Words may be spelled top to bottom, bottom to top, right to left, left to right, or diagonally.

```
S  U  D  O  R  I  F  E  R  O  U  S  V  K  R
E  J  U  Q  U  E  S  T  E  C  N  O  H  Y  U
I  S  J  L  M  E  L  A  N  O  C  Y  T  E  H
R  I  M  U  E  N  O  T  I  R  E  P  H  S  B
O  M  K  N  V  A  S  T  R  L  A  N  U  G  O
T  R  G  U  F  G  A  U  C  E  G  O  V  W  D
A  E  A  L  P  R  D  I  O  N  T  F  D  R  N
L  D  V  A  D  M  L  C  P  D  H  S  L  Z  F
I  I  N  Y  N  L  R  L  A  M  E  N  I  R  E
P  P  H  Q  O  N  E  U  X  R  R  F  E  L  G
E  E  Z  F  J  U  M  Y  O  U  U  O  C  C  B
D  Z  P  E  R  J  Y  U  V  F  C  I  I  E  O
G  J  S  I  W  J  S  K  C  D  T  N  O  Z  C
C  O  S  M  Z  M  F  I  B  U  G  U  X  O  J
X  Y  P  M  E  I  W  E  C  V  S  U  G  B  I
```

Apocrine	Epidermis	Mucus
Blister	Follicle	Peritoneum
Cuticle	Lanugo	Pleurisy
Dehydration	Lunula	Serous
Depilatories	Melanocyte	Sudoriferous

DID YOU KNOW?

Because the dead cells of the epidermis are constantly being worn and washed away, we get a new outer skin layer every 27 days.

SKIN/BODY MEMBRANES

Fill in the crossword puzzle.

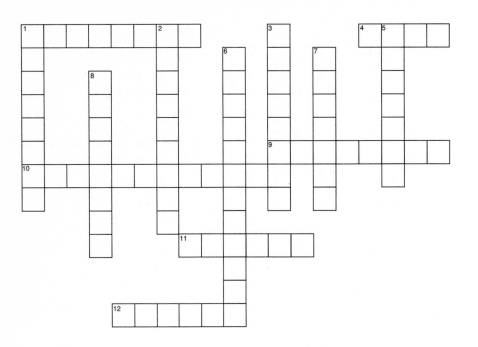

ACROSS

1. Inflammation of the serous membrane that lines the chest and covers the lungs
4. Cutaneous
9. Membrane that lines joint spaces
10. "Goose pimples" (two words)
11. Cushionlike sacs found between moving body parts
12. Deeper of the two primary skin layers

DOWN

1. Forms the lining of serous body cavities
2. Oil gland
3. Bluish-gray color of skin due to decreased oxygen
5. Tough waterproof substance that protects body from excess fluid loss
6. Sweat gland
7. Brown pigment
8. Covers the surface of organs found in serous body cavities

CHECK YOUR KNOWLEDGE

Multiple Choice

Circle the correct answer.

1. What is the type of serous membrane that covers organs that is found in all body cavities called?
    A. Visceral
    B. Pleural
    C. Parietal
    D. Synovial

2. Which of the following statements about synovial membranes is true?
    A. They are classified as epithelial.
    B. They line joints.
    C. They contain a parietal layer.
    D. All of the above are true.

3. Which of the following statements abut hair follicles is true?
    A. Arrector pili muscles are associated with them.
    B. Sudoriferous glands empty into them.
    C. They arise directly from the epidermis layer of skin.
    D. All of the above are true.

4. Which of the following statements about apocrine glands is true?
    A. They can be classified as sudoriferous.
    B. They are found primarily in armpit and genital regions.
    C. They secrete a thick substance that has a strong odor associated with it.
    D. All of the above are true.

5. Which of the following, if any, is *not* found in the dermis layer of the skin?
    A. Nerves
    B. Melanin
    C. Blood vessels
    D. All of the above are found in the dermis.

6. What characterizes second-degree burns?
    A. Blisters
    B. Swelling
    C. Severe pain
    D. All of the above

7. Blackheads can result from the blockage of which of the following glands?
    A. Lacrima
    B. Sebaceous
    C. Ceruminous
    D. Sudoriferous

8. Keratin is found in which layer of the skin?
    A. Dermis
    B. Epidermis
    C. Subcutaneous
    D. Serous

9. What is the fold of skin that hides the root of a nail called?
    A. Lunula
    B. Body
    C. Cuticle
    D. Papillae

10. Which of the following is *not* an important function of the skin?
    A. Sense organ activity
    B. Absorption
    C. Protection
    D. Temperature regulation

Matching

Select the most correct answer from column B for each statement in column A. (Only one answer is correct.)

Column A

_____ 11.   Melanin

_____ 12.   Epithelial membrane

_____ 13.   Pacinian corpuscle

_____ 14.   Sebaceous

_____ 15.   Waterproofing

_____ 16.   Hair

_____ 17.   Lunula

_____ 18.   Connective tissue membrane

_____ 19.   Dermal papillae

_____ 20.   Sudoriferous

Column B

A. Fingerprint

B. Skin receptor

C. Brown pigment

D. Pleura

E. Synovial membrane

F. Perspiration

G. Oil

H. Follicle

I. Keratin

J. Little moon

Completion

Complete the following using the terms below.

A. Skin

B. Eccrine sweat glands

C. Peritonitis

D. Mucous

E. Epidermis

F. Fourth-degree burns

G. Pleurisy

H. Sebaceous

I. Hair follicles

J. Receptors

_____ 21.   Which glands secrete oil or sebum for hair and skin?

_____ 22.   The first line of defense for the body is the _____.

_____ 23.   These glands work throughout the body, helping to regulate body heat.

_____ 24.   This burn extends below the subcutaneous tissue to muscle or bone.

_____ 25.   Hair growth requires epidermal, tubelike structures called _____.

_____ 26.   The outermost and thinnest primary layer of skin is _____.

_____ 27.   A condition that involves inflammation of the serous membranes lining the chest cavity and covering the lungs is called _____.

_____ 28.   This membrane lines body surfaces that open directly to the exterior of the body and produces mucus.

_____ 29.   Specialized nerve endings that make it possible for skin to act as a sense organ are called _____.

_____ 30.   A condition in which the serous membranes, which line the abdominal cavity and abdominal organs, are inflamed.

LONGITUDINAL SECTION OF THE SKIN

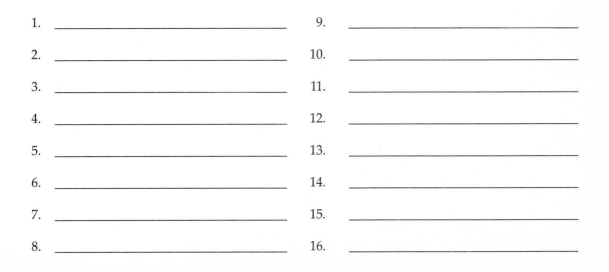

1. _____   9. _____

2. _____   10. _____

3. _____   11. _____

4. _____   12. _____

5. _____   13. _____

6. _____   14. _____

7. _____   15. _____

8. _____   16. _____

"RULE OF NINES" FOR ESTIMATING SKIN SURFACE BURNED

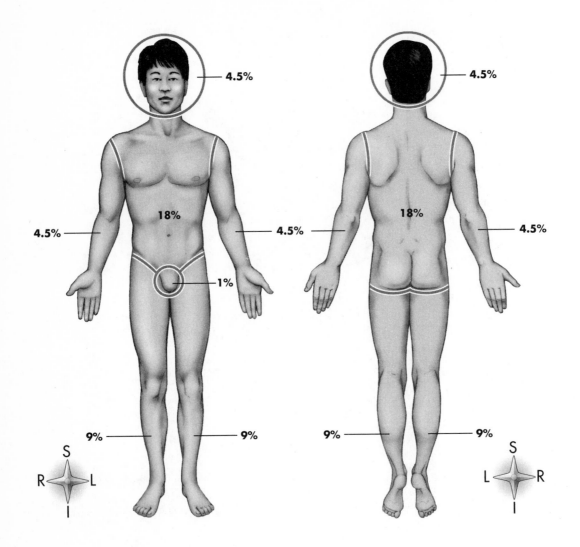

CHAPTER 7

The Skeletal System

How strange we would look without our skeleton! It is the skeleton that provides us with the rigid, supportive framework that gives shape to our bodies. But this is just the beginning, because the skeleton also protects the organs beneath it, maintains homeostasis of blood calcium, produces blood cells, and assists the muscular system in providing movement for us.

After reviewing the microscopic structure of bone and cartilage, you will understand how skeletal tissues are formed, their differences, and their importance in the human body. Your microscopic investigation will make the study of this system easier as you logically progress from this view to macroscopic bone formation and growth and visualize the structure of long bones.

The skeleton is divided into two main divisions: the axial skeleton and the appendicular skeleton. All of the 206 bones of the human body may be classified into one of these two areas. Although we can divide them neatly by this system, there are subtle differences that exist between a man's and a woman's skeleton. These structural differences provide us with insight to the functional differences between men and women.

Three types of joints exist in the body. They are synarthrosis, amphiarthrosis, and diarthrosis. It is important to have a knowledge of these joints to understand how movement is facilitated by articulations.

TOPICS FOR REVIEW

Before progressing to Chapter 8, you should familiarize yourself with the functions of the skeletal system, the structure and function of bone and cartilage, bone formation and growth, and the types of joints found in the body. Additionally, your understanding of the skeletal system should include identification of the two major subdivisions of the skeleton, the bones found in each area, and any differences that exist between a man's and a woman's skeleton. Your study should conclude with a review of the major skeletal disorders.

FUNCTIONS OF THE SKELETAL SYSTEM
TYPES OF BONES
STRUCTURE OF LONG BONES

Fill in the blanks.

1. There are _____ types of bones.

2. The _____ _____ is the hollow area inside the diaphysis of a bone.

3. A thin layer of cartilage covering each epiphysis is the _____
    _____.

4. The _____ lines the medullary cavity of long bones.

5. _____ is used to describe the process of blood cell formation.

6. Blood cell formation is a vital process carried on in _____
    _____ _____.

7. The _____ is a strong fibrous membrane that covers a long bone except
    at joint surfaces.

8. Bones may be classified by shape. Those shapes include _____,
    _____, _____, and
    _____.

9. Bones serve as a safety-deposit box for _____, a vital substance re-
    quired for normal nerve and muscle function.

10. As muscles contract and shorten, they pull on bones and thereby _____
    them.

> *If you have had difficulty with this section, review pages 180-183.*

MICROSCOPIC STRUCTURE OF BONE AND CARTILAGE

Match the term on the left with the proper selection on the right.

Group A

_____ 11. Trabeculae   A. Outer covering of bone
_____ 12. Compact   B. Dense bone tissue
_____ 13. Spongy   C. Fibers embedded in a firm gel
_____ 14. Periosteum   D. Needle-like threads of spongy bone
_____ 15. Cartilage   E. Ends of long bones

Group B

_____ 16. Osteocytes   A. Connect lacunae
_____ 17. Canaliculi   B. Cartilage cells
_____ 18. Lamellae   C. Structural unit of compact bone
_____ 19. Chondrocytes   D. Bone cells
_____ 20. Haversian system   E. Ring of bone

> *If you have had difficulty with this section, review pages 183-185.*

BONE FORMATION AND GROWTH

If the statement is true, write "T" in the answer blank. If the statement is false, correct the statement by circling the incorrect term and inserting the correct term in the answer blank.

_____ 21. When the skeleton forms in a baby before birth, it consists of cartilage and
                             fibrous structures.

_____ 22. The diaphyses are the ends of the bone.

_____ 23. Bone-forming cells are known as *osteoclasts*.

_____ 24. It is the combined action of osteoblasts and osteoclasts that sculpts bones into
                             their adult shapes.

_____ 25. The point of articulation between the epiphysis and diaphysis of a growing long bone is susceptible to injury if over-stressed.

_____ 26. The epiphyseal plate can be seen in both external and cutaway views of an adult long bone.

_____ 27. The shaft of a long bone is known as the _articulation_.

_____ 28. Cartilage in the newborn becomes bone when it is replaced with calcified bone matrix deposited by osteoblasts.

_____ 29. When epiphyseal cartilage becomes bone, growth begins.

_____ 30. The epiphyseal cartilage is visible, if present, on x-ray films.

▶ _If you have had difficulty with this section, review pages 185-187._

DIVISIONS OF SKELETON

Circle the correct answer.

31. Which of the following is/are _not_ a part of the axial skeleton?
    A. Scapula
    B. Cranial bones
    C. Vertebra
    D. Ribs
    E. Sternum

32. Which one of the following is _not_ a cranial bone?
    A. Frontal
    B. Parietal
    C. Occipital
    D. Lacrimal
    E. Sphenoid

33. Which of the following is _not_ correct?
    A. A baby is born with a straight spine.
    B. In the adult, the sacral and thoracic curves are convex.
    C. The normal curves of the adult spine provide greater strength than a straight spine.
    D. A curved structure has more strength than a straight one of the same size and materials.

34. True ribs:
    A. Attach to the cartilage of other ribs
    B. Do not attach to the sternum
    C. Attach directly to the sternum without cartilage
    D. Attach directly to the sternum by means of cartilage

35. The bone that runs along the lateral side of your forearm is the:
    A. Humerus
    B. Ulna
    C. Radius
    D. Tibia

36. The shinbone is also known as the:
    A. Fibula
    B. Femur
    C. Tibia
    D. Ulna

37. The bones in the palm of the hand are called:
    A. Metatarsals
    B. Tarsals
    C. Carpals
    D. Metacarpals

38. Which one of the following is _not_ a bone of the upper extremity?
    A. Radius
    B. Clavicle
    C. Humerus
    D. Ilium

39. The heel bone is known as the:
    A. Calcaneus
    B. Talus
    C. Metatarsal
    D. Phalanges

40. The mastoid process is part of which bone?
    A. Parietal
    B. Temporal
    C. Occipital
    D. Frontal

41. When a baby learns to walk, which area of the spine becomes concave?
    A. Lumbar
    B. Thoracic
    C. Cervical
    D. Coccyx

42. Which bone is the "funny" bone?
    A. Radius
    B. Ulna
    C. Humerus
    D. Carpal

43. There are how many pair of true ribs?
    A. 14
    B. 7
    C. 5
    D. 3

44. The 27 bones in the wrist and the hand allow
    for more:
    A. Strength
    B. Dexterity
    C. Protection
    D. Red blood cell products

45. The longest bone in the body is the:
    A. Tibia
    B. Fibula
    C. Femur
    D. Humerus

46. Distally, the _____ articulates with the
    patella.
    A. Femur
    B. Fibula
    C. Tibia
    D. Humerus

47. These bones form the cheek bones.
    A. Mandible
    B. Palatine
    C. Maxillary
    D. Zygomatic

48. In a child, there are five of these bones. In an
    adult, they are fused into one.
    A. Pelvic
    B. Lumbar vertebrae
    C. Sacrum
    D. Carpals

49. The spinal cord enters the cranium through a
    large hole (foramen magnum) in this bone.
    A. Temporal
    B. Parietal
    C. Occipital
    D. Sphenoid

Circle the one that does not belong.

50. Cervical	Thoracic	Coxal	Coccyx
51. Pelvic girdle	Ankle	Wrist	Axial
52. Frontal	Occipital	Maxilla	Sphenoid
53. Scapula	Pectoral girdle	Ribs	Clavicle
54. Malleus	Vomer	Incus	Stapes
55. Ulna	Ilium	Ischium	Pubis
56. Carpal	Phalanges	Metacarpal	Ethmoid
57. Ethmoid	Parietal	Occipital	Nasal
58. Anvil	Atlas	Axis	Cervical

▶ _If you have had difficulty with this section, review pages 187-204._

DIFFERENCES BETWEEN A MAN'S AND A WOMAN'S SKELETON

Choose the correct answer.

A. Male   B. Female

_____ 59. Funnel-shaped pelvis

_____ 60. Broader-shaped pelvis

_____ 61. Wider pubic angle

_____ 62. Larger

_____ 63. Wider pelvic inlet

▶ *If you have had difficulty with this section, review pages 204-205.*

BONE MARKINGS

From the choices given, match the bone with its identification marking. Answer choices may be used more than once.

A. Mastoid
B. Pterygoid process
C. Foramen magnum
D. Sella turcica
E. Mental foramen
F. Conchae
G. Xiphoid process

H. Glenoid cavity
I. Olecranon process
J. Ischium
K. Acetabulum
L. Symphysis pubis
M. Ilium
N. Greater trochanter

O. Medial malleolus
P. Calcaneus
Q. Acromion process
R. Frontal sinuses
S. Condyloid process
T. Tibial tuberosity

_____ 64. Occipital

_____ 65. Sternum

_____ 66. Coxal

_____ 67. Femur

_____ 68. Ulna

_____ 69. Temporal

_____ 70. Tarsals

_____ 71. Sphenoid

_____ 72. Ethmoid

_____ 73. Scapula

_____ 74. Tibia

_____ 75. Frontal

_____ 76. Mandible

▶ *If you have had difficulty with this section, review pages 190, 196, 200, and 203.*

JOINTS (ARTICULATIONS)

Circle the correct answer.

77. Freely movable joints are (amphiarthroses or diarthroses).

78. The sutures in the skull are (synarthrotic or amphiarthrotic) joints.

79. All (diarthrotic or amphiarthrotic) joints have a joint capsule, a joint cavity, and a layer of cartilage over the ends of the two joining bones.

80. (Ligaments or tendons) grow out of periosteum and attach two bones together.

81. The (articular cartilage or epiphyseal cartilage) absorbs jolts.

82. Gliding joints are the (least movable or most movable) of the diarthrotic joints.

83. The knee is the (largest or smallest) joint.

84. Hinge joints allow motion in (2 or 4) directions.

85. The saddle joint at the base of each of our thumbs allows for greater (strength or mobility).

86. When you rotate your head, you are using a (gliding or pivot) joint.

▶ *If you have had difficulty with this section, review pages 205-212.*

SKELETAL DISORDERS

Fill in the blanks.

87. _____ is an imaging technique that allows a physician to examine the internal structure of a joint without the use of extensive surgery.

88. One of the most common skeletal tumors and one of the most rapidly fatal is _____.

89. A common bone disease characterized by excessive loss of calcified matrix and collagenous fiber is _____.

90. A metabolic disorder involving mineral loss in bones is _____.

91. A metabolic disorder that is often asymptomatic and affects older adults is _____.

92. The general name for bacterial infections of bone and marrow tissue is _____.

93. Closed fractures, also known as _____ _____, do not pierce the skin.

94. _____ _____ are breaks that produce many fragments.

95. The most common noninflammatory joint disease is _____ or _____, _____ _____.

96. Three major types of arthritis are _____, _____, and _____.

97. One form of infectious arthritis, _____ _____, was identified in 1975 in Connecticut and has since spread across the continent.

▶ *If you have had difficulty with this section, review pages 212-219.*

UNSCRAMBLE THE BONES

98. **E T V E R R B A E**

99. **B P S U I**

100. **S C A L U P A**

101. **I M D B A L N E**

102. **A P N H G A E L S**

Take the circled letters, unscramble them, and fill in the statement.

What the fat lady wore to the ball.

103.

APPLYING WHAT YOU KNOW

104. Mrs. Perine had advanced cancer of the bone. As the disease progressed, Mrs. Perine required several blood transfusions throughout her therapy. She asked the doctor one day to explain the necessity for the transfusions. What explanation might the doctor give to Mrs. Perine?

105. Dr. Kennedy, an orthopedic surgeon, called the admissions office of the hospital and advised that he would be admitting a patient in the next hour with an epiphyseal fracture. Without any other information, the patient is assigned to the pediatric ward. What prompted this assignment?

106. Mrs. Van Skiver, age 60, noticed when she went in for her physical examination that she was a half inch shorter than she was on her last visit. Dr. Veazey suggested she begin a regimen of dietary supplements of calcium, vitamin D, and a prescription for sex hormone therapy. What bone disease did Dr. Veazey suspect?

107. Mr. Ferber was moving and experienced severe sharp pain in his lower back while lifting some boxes. The pain was not relieved by traditional home remedies or pain medication. He finally sought the advice of a physician after being unable to relieve the pain for 48 hours. What might be a possible diagnosis?

108. Word Find

Can you find the 14 terms from this chapter that are listed below? Words may be spelled top to bottom, bottom to top, right to left, left to right, or diagonally.

```
A R T I C U L A T I O N N U T
M M L T N I N G U I H J N C G
P R P E R I O S T E U M A N B
H V P G U A T B M E O P R F G
I N V R N O B O F S M H X E R
A G J O A J P E T O E O H T Q
R U R B X O E E C A S G I S B
T S S Y I M O Q N U O O L X Q
H J I E A B P U N Q L E Q K S
R I S I L U C I L A N A C X R
O I N A M A S Q M A Q K E C T
S T S A L C O E T S O U I D G
E T S Y F W L N M P U F N U F
S B H Q H L O U S A R X I T V
R P M P A F M G X K D S L G A
```

Amphiarthroses	Fontanels	Osteoclasts
Articulation	Hemopoiesis	Periosteum
Axial	Lacunae	Sinus
Canaliculi	Lamella	Trabeculae
Compact	Osteoblasts	

DID YOU KNOW?

The bones of the hands and feet make up more than half of the total 206 bones of the body.

Approximately 25 million Americans have osteoporosis. Four out of five are women.

The bones of the middle ear are mature at birth.

SKELETAL SYSTEM

Fill in the crossword puzzle.

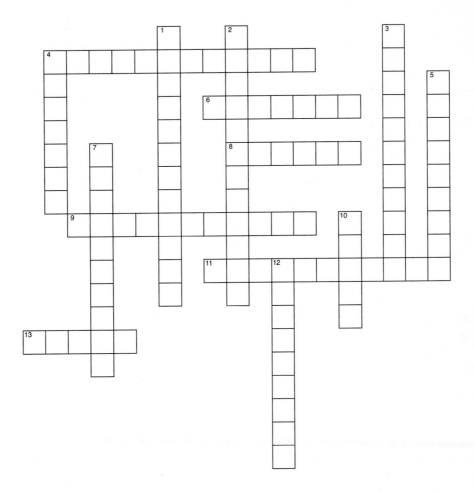

ACROSS

4. Cartilage cells
6. Spaces in bones where osteocytes are found
8. Chest
9. Freely movable joints
11. Process of blood cell formation
13. Space inside cranial bone

DOWN

1. Joint
2. Suture joints
3. Bone-absorbing cells
4. Type of bone
5. Ends of long bones
7. Covers long bone except at its joint surfaces
10. Division of skeleton
12. Bone cell

CHECK YOUR KNOWLEDGE

Multiple Choice

Circle the correct answer.

1. Which of the following statements concerning the ribs is true?
   A. The first seven pairs attach to the sternum by cartilage.
   B. The last four pairs are called *floating ribs* because they are free in the front.
   C. The eighth, ninth, and tenth pairs do not move because they are not attached to the sternum.
   D. All of the above statements concerning the ribs are true.

2. Which is the largest bone in the lower extremities?
   A. Humerus
   B. Ulna
   C. Femur
   D. Radius

3. Of what is yellow bone marrow primarily made?
   A. Fatty tissue
   B. Blood cells
   C. Epithelial tissue
   D. Fibrous tissue

4. Which of the following statements regarding the female pelvis is *not* true?
   A. Its shape can be described as broader, shallower, and basinlike when compared to that of the male.
   B. Its pelvic inlet, or brim, is usually wider than that of the male.
   C. Its individual hipbones are usually larger and heavier than those of the male.
   D. All of the above statements are true.

5. Which of the following statements are true about the normal curves of the spine (two concave and two convex)?
   A. They are present at birth.
   B. They extend from the skull to the bottom of the ribcage.
   C. They give the spine strength to support the weight of the rest of the body.
   D. All of the above are true.

6. Which of the following statements regarding diarthroses is *not* true?
   A. They contain a synovial membrane that secretes a lubricating fluid called *synovial fluid*.
   B. A diarthrotic joint may permit flexion, extension, abduction, adduction, or rotation.
   C. These joints make up the largest category of body joints.
   D. All of the above statements are true.

7. Which of the following bones are components of the axial skeletal system?
   A. Ilium, ethmoid, clavicle
   B. Ulna, palatine, occipital
   C. Sacrum, vomer, sphenoid
   D. Scapula, patella, fibula

8. Which of the following bones is *not* classified as a cranial bone?
   A. Sphenoid
   B. Parietal
   C. Palatine
   D. Temporal

9. Which of the following statements characterizes the skeleton of a growing child?
   A. Epiphyses are separated from diaphyses by a layer of cartilage.
   B. Osteoblasts deposit calcium in the gel-like matrix of cartilage.
   C. The periosteum is present.
   D. All of the above statements characterize the skeleton of a growing child.

10. What are the joints between the cranial bones called?
    A. Synarthroses
    B. Diarthroses
    C. Amphiarthroses
    D. All of the above

Matching

Select the most correct answer from column B for each statement in column A. (Only one answer is correct.)

Column A

_____ 11. Diarthroses

_____ 12. Spongy bone

_____ 13. Synarthrosis

_____ 14. Foramen magnum

_____ 15. Calcaneus

_____ 16. Chondrocyte

_____ 17. Compact bone

_____ 18. Ethmoid

_____ 19. Coxal

_____ 20. Hemopoiesis

Column B

A. Haversian canal

B. Trabeculae

C. Perpendicular plate

D. Red bone marrow

E. Tarsal

F. Ilium

G. Synovial fluid

H. Cartilage

I. Suture

J. Occipital bone

LONGITUDINAL SECTION OF LONG BONE

1. _____

2. _____

3. _____

4. _____

5. _____

6. _____

7. _____

8. _____

9. _____

10. _____

11. _____

ANTERIOR VIEW OF SKELETON

1. _____
2. _____
3. _____
4. _____
5. _____
6. _____
7. _____
8. _____
9. _____
10. _____
11. _____
12. _____
13. _____
14. _____
15. _____
16. _____
17. _____
18. _____
19. _____
20. _____
21. _____
22. _____
23. _____
24. _____
25. _____
26. _____
27. _____
28. _____
29. _____
30. _____

POSTERIOR VIEW OF SKELETON

1. _____

2. _____

3. _____

4. _____

5. _____

6. _____

7. _____

8. _____

9. _____

10. _____

11. _____

12. _____

13. _____

14. _____

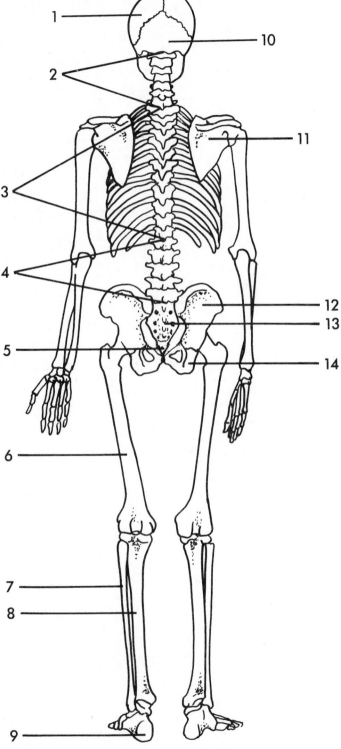

SKULL VIEWED FROM THE RIGHT SIDE

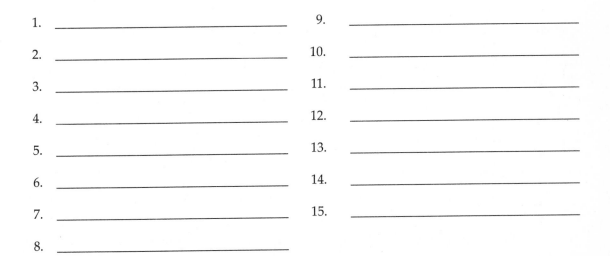

1. _____   9. _____

2. _____   10. _____

3. _____   11. _____

4. _____   12. _____

5. _____   13. _____

6. _____   14. _____

7. _____   15. _____

8. _____

SKULL VIEWED FROM THE FRONT

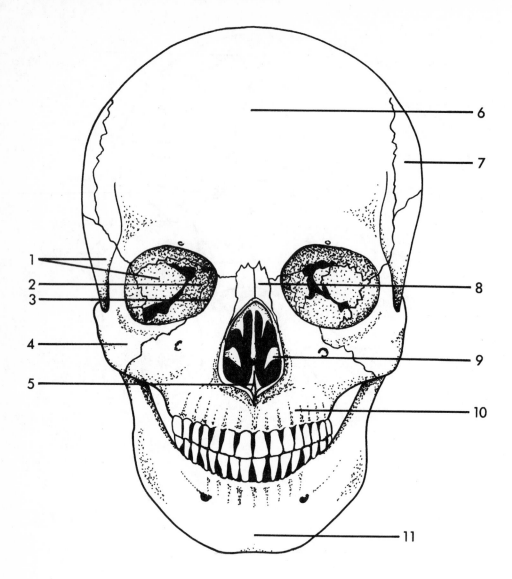

1. _____   7. _____

2. _____   8. _____

3. _____   9. _____

4. _____   10. _____

5. _____   11. _____

6. _____

STRUCTURE OF A DIARTHROTIC JOINT

1. _____

2. _____

3. _____

4. _____

5. _____

6. _____

7. _____

8. _____

9. _____

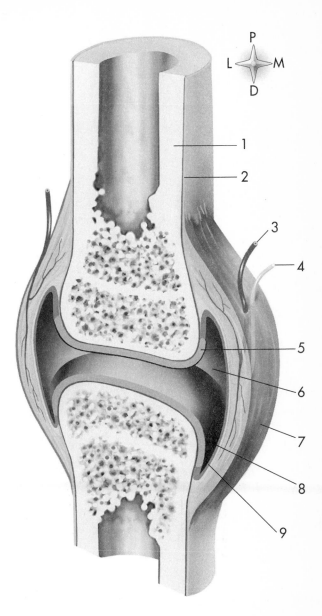

CHAPTER 8

The Muscular System

The muscular system is often referred to as the "power system," and rightfully so, because it is this system that provides the force necessary to move the body and perform organic functions. Just as an automobile relies on the engine to provide motion, the body depends on the muscular system to perform both voluntary and involuntary types of movement. Walking, breathing, and the digestion of food are but a few examples of body functions that require the healthy performance of the muscular system.

Although this system has several functions, the primary purpose is to provide movement or power. Muscles produce power by contracting. The ability of a large muscle or muscle group to contract depends on the ability of microscopic muscle fibers to contract within the larger muscle. An understanding of these microscopic muscle fibers will assist you as you progress in your study to the larger muscles and muscle groups.

Muscle contractions may be one of several types: isotonic, isometric, twitch, or tetanic. When skeletal or voluntary muscles contract, they provide us with a variety of motions. Flexion, extension, abduction, adduction, and rotation are examples of these movements that provide us with both strength and agility.

Muscles must be used to keep the body healthy and in good condition. Scientific evidence keeps pointing to the fact that the proper use and exercise of muscles may prolong longevity. An understanding of the structure and function of the muscular system may, therefore, add quality and quantity to our lives.

TOPICS FOR REVIEW

Before progressing to Chapter 9, you should familiarize yourself with the structure and function of the three major types of muscle tissue. Your review should include the microscopic structure of skeletal muscle tissue, how a muscle is stimulated, the major types of skeletal muscle contractions, and the skeletal muscle groups. Your study should conclude with an understanding of the types of movements produced by skeletal muscle contractions and the major muscular disorders.

MUSCLE TISSUE

Select the correct term from the choices provided and insert the letter(s) in the answer blank.

A. Skeletal muscle   B. Cardiac muscle   C. Smooth muscle

_____ 1.   Striated

_____ 2.   Cells branch frequently

_____ 3.   Moves food into the stomach

_____ 4.   Nonstriated

_____ 5.   Voluntary

_____ 6.   Keeps blood circulating through its vessels

_____ 7.   Involuntary

_____ 8.   Attaches to bone

_____ 9.   Hollow internal organs

_____ 10.   Maintenance of normal blood pressure

▶ *If you have had difficulty with this section, review pages 228-231.*

STRUCTURE OF SKELETAL MUSCLES

Match the term on the left with the proper selection on the right.

_____ 11.	Origin	A.	The muscle unit excluding the ends
_____ 12.	Insertion	B.	Attachment to the more movable bone
_____ 13.	Body	C.	Fluid-filled sacs
_____ 14.	Tendons	D.	Attachment to more stationary bone
_____ 15.	Bursae	E.	Anchor muscles to bones

MICROSCOPIC STRUCTURE

_____ 16.	Muscle fibers	A.	Protein that forms thick myofilaments
_____ 17.	Actin	B.	Basic functional unit of skeletal muscle
_____ 18.	Sarcomere	C.	Protein that forms thin myofilaments
_____ 19.	Myosin	D.	Microscopic threadlike structures found in skeletal muscle fibers
_____ 20.	Myofilaments	E.	Specialized contractile cells of muscle tissue

▶ *If you have had difficulty with this section, review pages 231-233.*

FUNCTIONS OF SKELETAL MUSCLE

Fill in the blanks.

21. Muscles move bones by _____ on them.

22. As a rule, only the _____ bone moves.

23. The _____ bone moves toward the _____ bone.

24. Of all the muscles contracting simultaneously, the one mainly responsible for producing a particular movement is called the _____ _____ for that movement.

25. As prime movers contract, other muscles called _____ relax.

26. The biceps brachii is the prime mover during flexing, and the brachialis is its helper or _____ muscle.

27. We are able to maintain our body position because of a specialized type of skeletal muscle contraction called _____ _____.

28. _____ _____ maintains body posture by counteracting the pull of gravity.

29. A decrease in temperature, a condition known as _____, will drastically affect cellular activity and normal body function.

30. Energy required to produce a muscle contraction is obtained from _____.

▶ *If you have had difficulty with this section, review pages 233-234.*

FATIGUE
ROLE OF OTHER BODY SYSTEMS
MOTOR UNIT
MUSCLE STIMULUS

If the statement is true, write "T" on the answer blank. If the statement is false, correct the statement by circling the incorrect term and inserting the correct term in the answer blank.

_____ 31. The point of contact between the nerve ending and the muscle fiber is called a *motor neuron*.

_____ 32. A motor neuron together with the cells it innervates is called a *motor unit*.

_____ 33. If muscle cells are stimulated repeatedly without adequate periods of rest, the strength of the muscle contraction will decrease resulting in fatigue.

_____ 34. The depletion of oxygen in muscle cells during vigorous and prolonged exercise is known as *fatigue*.

_____ 35. An adequate stimulus will contract a muscle cell completely because of the "must" theory.

_____ 36. When oxygen supplies run low, muscle cells produce ATP and other waste products during contraction.

_____ 37. In a laboratory setting, a single muscle fiber can be isolated and subjected to stimuli of varying intensities so that it can be studied.

_____ 38. The minimal level of stimulation required to cause a fiber to contract is called the *threshold stimulus*.

_____ 39. Smooth muscles bring about movements by pulling on bones across movable joints.

_____ 40. A nervous system disorder that shuts off impulses to certain skeletal muscles may result in paralysis.

TYPES OF SKELETAL MUSCLE CONTRACTION

Circle the correct answer.

41. When a muscle does not shorten and no movement results, the contraction is:
    A. Isometric
    B. Isotonic
    C. Twitch
    D. Tetanic

42. Walking is an example of which type of contraction?
    A. Isometric
    B. Isotonic
    C. Twitch
    D. Tetanic

43. Pushing against a wall is an example of which type of contraction?
    A. Isotonic
    B. Isometric
    C. Twitch
    D. Tetanic

44. Endurance training is also known as:
    A. Isometrics
    B. Hypertrophy
    C. Aerobic training
    D. Strength training

45. Benefits of regular exercise include all of the following *except*:
    A. Improved lung functioning
    B. More efficient heart
    C. Less fatigue
    D. Atrophy

46. Twitch contractions easily can be seen:
    A. In isolated muscles prepared for research
    B. In a great deal of normal muscle activity
    C. During resting periods
    D. None of the above

47. Individual contractions "melt" together to produce a sustained contraction or:
    A. Twitch
    B. Tetanus
    C. Isotonic response
    D. Isometric response

48. In most cases, isotonic contraction of muscle produces movement at a/an:
    A. Insertion
    B. Beginning
    C. Joint
    D. Bursa

49. Prolonged inactivity causes muscles to shrink in mass, a condition called:
    A. Hypertrophy
    B. Disuse atrophy
    C. Paralysis
    D. Muscle fatigue

50. Muscle hypertrophy can be best enhanced by a program of:
    A. Isotonic exercise
    B. Better posture
    C. High-protein diet
    D. Strength training

If you have had difficulty with this section, review pages 234-238.

SKELETAL MUSCLE GROUPS

Choose the proper function(s) for the muscles listed below and place the letter(s) in the answer blank.

A. Flexor   C. Abductor   E. Rotator
B. Extensor   D. Adductor   F. Dorsiflexor or plantar flexor

_____ 51. Deltoid
_____ 52. Tibialis anterior
_____ 53. Gastrocnemius
_____ 54. Biceps brachii
_____ 55. Gluteus medius

_____ 56. Soleus

_____ 57. Iliopsoas

_____ 58. Pectoralis major

_____ 59. Gluteus maximus

_____ 60. Triceps brachii

_____ 61. Sternocleidomastoid

_____ 62. Trapezius

_____ 63. Gracilis

▶ *If you have had difficulty with this section, review pages 238-245 and 249.*

TYPES OF MOVEMENTS PRODUCED BY SKELETAL MUSCLE CONTRACTIONS

Circle the correct answer.

64. A movement that makes the angle between two bones smaller is:
    A. Flexion
    B. Extension
    C. Abduction
    D. Adduction

65. Moving a part toward the midline is:
    A. Flexion
    B. Extension
    C. Abduction
    D. Adduction

66. Moving a part away from the midline is:
    A. Flexion
    B. Extension
    C. Abduction
    D. Adduction

67. When you move your head from side to side as in shaking your head "no" you are _____ a muscle group.
    A. Rotating
    B. Pronating
    C. Supinating
    D. Abducting

68. _____ occurs when you turn the palm of your hand from an anterior to posterior position.
    A. Dorsiflexion
    B. Plantar flexion
    C. Supination
    D. Pronation

69. Dorsiflexion refers to:
    A. Hand movements
    B. Eye movements
    C. Foot movements
    D. Head movements

▶ *If you have had difficulty with this section, review pages 245-249.*

MAJOR MUSCULAR DISORDERS

Circle the correct answer.

70. Muscle strains are characterized by (myalgia or fibromyositis).

71. Crush injuries can cause (hemoglobin or myoglobin) to accumulate in the blood and result in kidney failure.

72. A viral infection of the nerves that controls skeletal muscle movement is known as (poliomyelitis or muscular dystrophy).

73. (Muscular dystrophy or Myasthenia gravis) is a group of genetic diseases characterized by atrophy of skeletal muscle tissues.

74. (Muscular dystrophy or Myasthenia gravis) is an autoimmune disease in which the immune system attacks muscle cells at the neuromuscular junction.

 If you have had difficulty with this section, review pages 249-251.

APPLYING WHAT YOU KNOW

75. Casey noticed pain whenever she reached for anything in her cupboards. Her doctor told her that the small fluid-filled sacs in her shoulder were inflamed. What condition did Casey have?

76. The nurse was preparing an injection for Mrs. Tatakis. The amount to be given was 2 ml. What area of the body will the nurse most likely select for this injection?

77. Chris was playing football and pulled a band of fibrous connective tissue that attached a muscle to a bone. What is the common term for this tissue?

78. Word Find

Can you find the 25 muscle terms that are listed below? Words may be spelled top to bottom, bottom to top, right to left, left to right, or diagonally.

```
G  A  S  T  R  O  C  N  E  M  I  U  S  D  U
M  S  G  I  O  N  O  I  S  N  E  T  X  E  U
U  R  N  N  T  O  M  S  R  B  S  F  D  T  T
S  U  I  S  C  I  B  O  N  T  P  N  E  A  R
C  B  R  E  U  X  V  T  O  O  E  C  L  I  A
L  Q  T  R  D  E  C  O  D  A  C  M  T  R  P
E  T  S  T  B  L  M  N  N  V  I  E  O  T  E
X  F  M  I  A  F  Y  I  E  Y  B  N  I  S  Z
S  I  A  O  V  I  E  C  T  L  S  S  D  I  I
S  Y  H  N  S  S  R  O  T  A  T  O  R  G  U
U  A  M  G  A  R  H  P  A  I  D  J  N  R  S
E  H  A  T  R  O  P  H  Y  L  N  J  T  E  B
L  N  O  H  T  D  E  U  G  I  T  A  F  N  T
O  R  I  G  I  N  O  S  N  V  S  B  Z  Y  L
S  B  V  T  O  J  C  T  R  I  C  E  P  S  S
```

Abductor	Flexion	Soleus
Atrophy	Gastrocnemius	Striated
Biceps	Hamstrings	Synergist
Bursa	Insertion	Tendon
Deltoid	Isometric	Tenosynovitis
Diaphragm	Isotonic	Trapezius
Dorsiflexion	Muscle	Triceps
Extension	Origin	
Fatigue	Rotator	

DID YOU KNOW?

If all of your muscles pulled in one direction, you would have the power to move 25 tons.

THE MUSCULAR SYSTEM

Fill in the crossword puzzle.

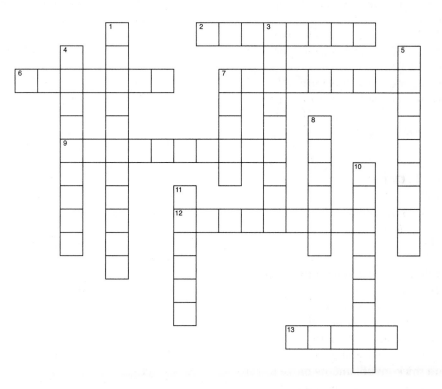

ACROSS	DOWN
2. Shaking your head "no"	1. Increase in size
6. Muscle shrinkage	3. Away from the body's midline
7. Toward the body's midline	4. Turning your palm from an anterior to posterior position
9. Produces movement opposite to prime movers	5. Attachment to the more movable bone
12. Movement that makes joint angles larger	7. Protein which composes myofilaments
13. Small fluid-filled sac between tendons and bones	8. Attachment to the more stationary bone
	10. Assists prime movers with movement
	11. Anchors muscles to bones

CHECK YOUR KNOWLEDGE

Multiple Choice

Circle the correct answer.

1. Which of the following statements about a motor unit is true?
   A. It consists of a muscle cell group and a motor neuron.
   B. The point of contact between the nerve ending and the muscle fiber is called the *neuromuscular junction*.
   C. Chemicals generate events within the muscle cell that result in contraction of the muscle cell.
   D. All of the above are true.

2. What is movement of a part away from the midline of the body called?
   A. Abduction
   B. Adduction
   C. Pronation
   D. Plantar flexion

3. According to the sliding filament theory of muscle contraction:
   A. Muscle fibers contain thin myofilaments made of a protein called *myosin*.
   B. Muscle fibers contain thick myofilaments made up of a protein called *actin*.
   C. Thin and thick myofilaments move toward each other to cause muscle contraction.
   D. All of the above are true.

4. Which of the following statements is true of the hamstring group of muscles?
   A. It includes the rectus femoris.
   B. It flexes the knee.
   C. It originates on the pubis.
   D. All of the above are true.

5. What happens if a given muscle cell is stimulated by a threshold stimulus?
   A. It shows an "all or none" response.
   B. It shows a tetanus response.
   C. It shows a subminimal response.
   D. None of the above is true.

6. Which of the following statements about oxygen debt is true?
   A. It is caused when excess oxygen is present in the environment.
   B. It causes lactic acid buildup and soreness in muscles.
   C. It can be replaced by slow, shallow breathing.
   D. All of the above are true.

7. What is a quick, jerky response of a given muscle to a single stimulus called?
   A. Isometric
   B. Lockjaw
   C. Tetanus
   D. Twitch

8. Which of the following statements about muscle atrophy is true?
   A. It decreases the size of a muscle.
   B. It increases the size of a muscle.
   C. Has no effect on muscle size.
   D. None of the above is true.

9. Which of the following occurs during isometric exercises?
   A. Muscle length remains the same.
   B. Muscle tension remains the same.
   C. Muscle length shortens.
   D. None of the above occurs.

10. Which of the following statements about skeletal muscle contraction is true?
    A. Its attachment to the more stationary bone is called its *origin*.
    B. Its attachment to the more moveable bone is called its *insertion*.
    C. Both A and B are true.
    D. None of the above is true.

True/False

If the statement is true, write "T" on the answer blank. If the statement is false, correct the statement by circling the incorrect term and inserting the correct term in the answer blank.

_____ 11. When a part is moved toward the midline, it is called *adduction*.

_____ 12. An isometric contraction does not shorten or move a muscle.

_____ 13. Dorsiflexion occurs when you turn the palm of your hand from an anterior to a posterior position.

_____ 14. Exercise may cause an increase in muscle size called *atrophy*.

_____ 15. Isotonic contraction is an example of a contraction used while walking.

_____ 16. If a muscle is overworked without sufficient rest, the result will be a decrease in muscle strength and fatigue.

_____ 17. A bone of insertion moves toward the bone of origin.

_____ 18. A condition in which the body temperature is drastically low is referred to as *hyperthermia*.

_____ 19. Tetanic contraction is caused by a series of rapid stimuli.

_____ 20. When the angle between two bones becomes smaller, it is called *extension*.

MUSCLES—ANTERIOR VIEW

1. _____

2. _____

3. _____

4. _____

5. _____

6. _____

7. _____

8. _____

9. _____

10. _____

11. _____

12. _____

13. _____

14. _____

15. _____

16. _____

17. _____

18. _____

MUSCLES—POSTERIOR VIEW

1. _____

2. _____

3. _____

4. _____

5. _____

6. _____

7. _____

8. _____

9. _____

10. _____

11. _____

12. _____

13. _____

Semitendinosus

9 { Biceps femoris

Semimembranosus

CHAPTER 9

The Nervous System

The nervous system organizes and coordinates the millions of impulses received each day to make communication with and enjoyment of our environment possible. The functioning unit of the nervous system is the neuron. Three types of neurons exist—sensory, motor, and interneurons—which are classified according to the direction in which they transmit impulses. Nerve impulses travel over routes made up of neurons and provide the rapid communication necessary for maintaining life. The central nervous system is made up of the spinal cord and brain. The spinal cord provides access to and from the brain by means of ascending and descending tracts. In addition, the spinal cord functions as the primary reflex center of the body. The brain consists of the brain stem, cerebellum, diencephalon, and cerebrum. These areas provide the extraordinary network necessary to receive, interpret, and respond to the simplest or most complex impulses.

While you concentrate on this chapter, your body is performing a multitude of functions. Fortunately for us, the beating of the heart, the digestion of food, breathing, and most of our other day-to-day processes do not require our supervision or thought. They function automatically, and the division of the nervous system that regulates these functions is known as the *autonomic nervous system*. The autonomic nervous system consists of two divisions called the *sympathetic system* and the *parasympathetic system*. The sympathetic system functions as an emergency system and prepares us for "fight or flight." The parasympathetic system dominates control of many visceral effectors under normal everyday conditions. Together, these two divisions regulate the body's automatic functions in an effort to assist with the maintenance of homeostasis. Your understanding of this chapter will alert you to the complexity and functions of the nervous system and the "automatic pilot" of your body—the autonomic system.

TOPICS FOR REVIEW

Before progressing to Chapter 10, you should review the organs and divisions of the nervous system, the structure and function of the major types of cells in this system, the structure and function of a reflex arc, and the transmission of nerve impulses. Your study should include the anatomy and physiology of the brain and spinal cord and the nerves that extend from these two areas. Finally, an understanding of the autonomic nervous system, the specific functions of the subdivisions of this system, and the major disorders of the nervous system are necessary to complete the review of this chapter.

ORGANS AND DIVISIONS OF THE NERVOUS SYSTEM
CELLS OF THE NERVOUS SYSTEM
NERVES

Match the term on the left with the proper selection on the right.

Group A

_____ 1. Sense organ

_____ 2. Central nervous system

_____ 3. Peripheral nervous system

_____ 4. Autonomic nervous system

A. Subdivision of peripheral nervous system

B. Ear

C. Brain and spinal cord

D. Nerves that extend to the outlying parts of the body

Group B

_____ 5. Dendrite

_____ 6. Schwann cell

_____ 7. Motor neuron

_____ 8. Nodes of Ranvier

_____ 9. Fascicles

_____ 10. Epineurium

A. Indentations between adjacent Schwann cells

B. Branching projection of neuron

C. Also known as *efferent*

D. Forms myelin outside the CNS

E. Tough sheath that covers the whole nerve

F. Groups of wrapped axons

CELLS OF NERVOUS SYSTEM
NERVES

Select the best choice for the following words and insert the correct letter in the answer blank.

A. Neurons   B. Neuroglia

_____ 11. Axon

_____ 12. Supporting cells

_____ 13. Astrocytes

_____ 14. Sensory

_____ 15. Conduct impulses

_____ 16. Forms the myelin sheath around central nerve fibers

_____ 17. Phagocytosis

_____ 18. Efferent

_____ 19. Multiple sclerosis

_____ 20. Neurilemma

▷ *If you have had difficulty with this section, review pages 260-267.*

REFLEX ARCS

Fill in the blanks.

21. The simplest kind of reflex arc is a _____

_____ _____.

22. Three-neuron arcs consist of all three kinds of neurons, _____,

_____, and _____

_____.

23. Impulse conduction in a reflex arc normally starts in _____.

24. A _____ is the microscopic space that separates the axon of one neuron
from the dendrites of another neuron.

25. A _____ is the response to impulse conduction over reflex arcs.

26. Contraction of a muscle that causes it to pull away from an irritating stimulus is known as the

_____ _____.

27. A _____ is a group of nerve-cell bodies located in the peripheral nervous system.

28. All _____ lie entirely within the gray matter of the central nervous system.

29. In a patellar reflex, the nerve impulses that reach the quadriceps muscle (the effector) result in the classic
_____ _____ response.

30. _____ _____ forms the H-shaped
inner core of the spinal cord.

▶ *If you have had difficulty with this section, review pages 267-270.*

NERVE IMPULSES
THE SYNAPSE

Circle the correct answer.

31. Nerve impulses (do or do not) continually race along every nerve cell's surface.

32. When a stimulus acts on a neuron, it (increases or decreases) the permeability of the stimulated point of
its membrane to sodium ions.

33. An inward movement of positive ions leaves a/an (lack or excess) of negative ions outside.

34. The plasma membrane of the (presynaptic or postsynaptic) neuron makes up a portion of the synapse.

35. A synaptic knob is a tiny bulge at the end of the (presynaptic or postsynaptic) neuron's axon.

36. Acetylcholine is an example of a (neurotransmitter or protein molecule receptor).

37. Neurotransmitters are chemicals that allow neurons to (communicate or reproduce) with one another.

38. Neurotransmitters are distributed (randomly or specifically) into groups of neurons.

39. Catecholamines may play a role in (sleep or reproduction).

40. Endorphins and enkephalins are neurotransmitters that inhibit conduction of (fear or pain) impulses.

▶ *If you have had difficulty with this section, review pages 270-274.*

CENTRAL NERVOUS SYSTEM
DIVISIONS OF THE BRAIN

Circle the correct answer.

41. The portion of the brain stem that joins the spinal cord to the brain is the:
    A. Pons
    B. Cerebellum
    C. Diencephalon
    D. Hypothalamus
    E. Medulla

42. Which one of the following is *not* a function of the brain stem?
    A. Conducts sensory impulses from the spinal cord to the higher centers of the brain.
    B. Conducts motor impulses from the cerebrum to the spinal cord.
    C. Controls heartbeat, respiration, and blood vessel diameter.
    D. Contains centers for speech and memory.

43. Which one of the following is *not* part of the diencephalon?
    A. Cerebrum
    B. Thalamus
    C. Pituitary gland
    D. Third ventricle gray matter

44. ADH is produced by the:
    A. Pituitary gland
    B. Medulla
    C. Mammillary bodies
    D. Third ventricle
    E. Hypothalamus

45. Which one of the following is *not* a function of the hypothalamus?
    A. It helps control the heart rate.
    B. It helps control the constriction and dilation of blood vessels.
    C. It helps control the contraction of the stomach and intestines.
    D. It produces hormones that control the release of certain anterior pituitary hormones.
    E. All of the above are functions of the hypothalamus.

46. Which one of the following parts of the brain helps in the association of sensations with emotions, as well as aiding in the arousal or alerting mechanism?
    A. Pons
    B. Hypothalamus
    C. Cerebellum
    D. Thalamus
    E. None of the above is correct

47. Which of the following is *not* true of the cerebrum?
    A. Its lobes correspond to the bones that lie over them.
    B. Its grooves are called *gyri*.
    C. Most of its gray matter lies on the surface of the cerebrum.
    D. Its outer region is called the *cerebral cortex*.
    E. Its two hemispheres are connected by a structure called the *corpus callosum*.

48. Which one of the following is *not* a function of the cerebrum?
    A. Willed movement
    B. Consciousness
    C. Memory
    D. Conscious awareness of sensations
    E. All of the above are functions of the cerebrum

49. The area of the cerebrum responsible for the perception of sound lies in the _____ lobe.
    A. Frontal
    B. Temporal
    C. Occipital
    D. Parietal

50. Visual perception is located in the _____ lobe.
    A. Frontal
    B. Temporal
    C. Parietal
    D. Occipital
    E. None of the above is correct

51. Which one of the following is *not* a function of the cerebellum?
    A. Maintains equilibrium
    B. Helps produce smooth, coordinated movements
    C. Helps maintain normal postures
    D. Associates sensations with emotions

52. Within the interior of the cerebrum are a few islands of gray matter known as:
    A. Fissures
    B. Basal ganglia
    C. Gyri
    D. Myelin

53. A cerebrovascular accident is commonly referred to as (a):
    A. Stroke
    B. Parkinson's disease
    C. Tumor
    D. Multiple sclerosis

54. Parkinson's disease is a disease of the:
    A. Myelin
    B. Axons
    C. Neuroglia
    D. Cerebral nuclei

55. The largest section of the brain is the:
    A. Cerebellum
    B. Pons
    C. Cerebrum
    D. Midbrain

▶ *If you have had difficulty with this section, review pages 274-278.*

BRAIN STUDIES

BRAIN DISORDERS

Select the best choice and insert the correct letter in the answer blank.

A. SPECT
B. MRI
C. CT
D. Hemiplegia
E. Cerebral palsy
F. EEG
G. Huntington's disease
H. CVA
I. Dementia
J. PET

_____ 56. Stroke

_____ 57. Paralysis of one side of the body

_____ 58. A crippling disease that involves permanent, nonprogressive damage to motor control areas of the brain

_____ 59. An imaging technique for the brain that involves scanning the head with a revolving x-ray generator

_____ 60. A scanning method that determines the functional characteristics of the brain by introducing a radioactive substance into the blood supply of the brain

_____ 61. Used to visualize blood flow in the brain

_____ 62. A scanning method that uses a magnetic field to induce brain tissues to emit radio waves

_____ 63. Measurement of electrical activity of the brain

_____ 64. Characteristic of Alzheimer's disease

_____ 65. Inherited disease characterized by chorea

▶ *If you have had difficulty with this section, review pages 278-282.*

SPINAL CORD

If the statement is true, write "T" on the answer blank. If the statement is false, correct the statement by circling the incorrect term and inserting the correct term in the answer blank.

_____ 66. The spinal cord is approximately 24 to 25 inches long.

_____ 67. The spinal cord ends at the bottom of the sacrum.

_____ 68. The extension of the meninges beyond the cord is convenient for performing CAT scans without danger of injuring the spinal cord.

_____ 69. Bundles of myelinated nerve fibers—dendrites—make up the white outer columns of the spinal cord.

_____ 70. Ascending tracts conduct impulses up the cord to the brain and descending tracts conduct impulses down the cord from the brain.

_____ 71. Tracts are functional organizations in that all of the axons that compose a tract serve several functions.

_____ 72. A loss of sensation caused by a spinal cord injury is called *paralysis*.

▶ *If you have had difficulty with this section, review pages 282-285.*

COVERINGS AND FLUID SPACES OF THE BRAIN AND SPINAL CORD

Circle the one that does not belong.

73. Meninges	Pia mater	Ventricles	Dura mater
74. Arachnoid	Middle layer	CSF	Cobweb-like
75. CSF	Ventricles	Subarachnoid space	Pia mater
76. Tough	Outer layer	Dura mater	Choroid plexus
77. Brain tumor	Subarachnoid space	CSF	Fourth lumbar vertebra

CRANIAL NERVES

78. Fill in the missing areas on the chart below.

NERVE		CONDUCT IMPULSES	FUNCTION
I		From nose to brain	Sense of smell
II	Optic	From eye to brain	
III	Oculomotor		Eye movements
IV		From brain to external eye muscles	Eye movements
V	Trigeminal	From skin and mucous membrane of head and from teeth to brain; also from brain to chewing muscles	

VI	Abducens		Eye movements
VII	Facial	From taste buds of tongue to brain; from brain to face muscles	
VIII		From ear to brain	Hearing; sense of balance
IX	Glossopharyngeal		Sensations of throat, taste, swallowing movements, secretion of saliva
X		From throat, larynx, and organs in thoracic and abdominal cavities to brain; also from brain to muscles of throat and abdominal cavities	Sensations of throat, larynx, and of thoracic and abdominal organs; swallowing, voice production, slowing of heartbeat, acceleration of peristalsis (gut movements)
XI	Accessory	From brain to certain shoulder and neck muscles	
XII		From brain to muscles of tongue	Tongue movements

▷ *If you have had difficulty with this section, review pages 285-289 and 291 Table 9-2.*

CRANIAL NERVES
SPINAL NERVES

Select the best choice for the following words and insert the correct letter in the answer blank.

A. Cranial nerves   B. Spinal nerves

_____ 79. 12 pairs

_____ 80. Dermatome

_____ 81. Vagus

_____ 82. Shingles

_____ 83. 31 pairs

_____ 84. Optic

_____ 85. C1

_____ 86. Plexus

▷ *If you have had difficulty with this section, review pages 289-292.*

AUTONOMIC NERVOUS SYSTEM

Match the term on the left with the proper selection on the right.

_____ 87. Autonomic nervous system

_____ 88. Autonomic neurons

_____ 89. Preganglionic neurons

_____ 90. Visceral effectors

_____ 91. Sympathetic nervous system

_____ 92. Somatic nervous system

A. Divisions of ANS

B. Tissues to which autonomic neurons conduct impulses

C. Voluntary actions

D. Regulates body's involuntary functions

E. Motor neurons that make up the ANS

F. Conduct impulses between the spinal cord and a ganglion

SYMPATHETIC NERVOUS SYSTEM
PARASYMPATHETIC NERVOUS SYSTEM

Circle the correct answer.

93. Dendrites and cell bodies of sympathetic pre-ganglionic neurons are located in the:
    A. Brain stem and sacral portion of the spinal cord
    B. Sympathetic ganglia
    C. Gray matter of the thoracic and upper lumbar segments of the spinal cord
    D. Ganglia close to effectors

94. Which of the following is *not* correct?
    A. Sympathetic preganglionic neurons have their cell bodies located in the lateral gray column of certain parts of the spinal cord.
    B. Sympathetic preganglionic axons pass along the dorsal root of certain spinal nerves.
    C. There are synapses within sympathetic ganglia.
    D. Sympathetic responses are usually widespread, involving many organs.

95. Another name for the parasympathetic nervous system is:
    A. Thoracolumbar
    B. Craniosacral
    C. Visceral
    D. ANS
    E. Cholinergic

96. Which statement is *not* correct?
    A. Sympathetic postganglionic neurons have their dendrites and cell bodies in sympathetic ganglia or collateral ganglia.
    B. Sympathetic ganglions are located in front of and at each side of the spinal column.
    C. Separate autonomic nerves distribute many sympathetic postganglionic axons to various internal organs.
    D. Very few sympathetic preganglionic axons synapse with postganglionic neurons.

97. Sympathetic stimulation usually results in a/an:
    A. Response by numerous organs
    B. Response by only one organ
    C. Increase in peristalsis
    D. Constriction of pupils

98. Parasympathetic stimulation frequently results in a/an:
    A. Response by only one organ
    B. Response by numerous organs
    C. Fight-or-flight syndrome
    D. Increase in heartbeat

Choose the correct answer and insert the letter in answer blanks.

A. Sympathetic control   B. Parasympathetic control

_____ 99. Constricts pupils

_____ 100. "Goose pimples"

_____ 101. Increases sweat secretion

_____ 102. Increases secretion of digestive juices

_____ 103. Constricts blood vessels

_____ 104. Slows heartbeat

_____ 105. Relaxes bladder

_____ 106. Increases epinephrine secretion

_____ 107. Increases peristalsis

_____ 108. Stimulates lens for near vision

▷ *If you have had difficulty with this section, review pages 292-297.*

AUTONOMIC NEUROTRANSMITTERS
AUTONOMIC NERVOUS SYSTEM AS A WHOLE

Fill in the blanks.

109. Sympathetic preganglionic axons release the neurotransmitter _____.

110. Axons that release norepinephrine are classified as _____ _____.

111. Axons that release acetylcholine are classified as _____ _____.

112. The function of the autonomic nervous system is to regulate the body's involuntary functions in ways that maintain or restore _____.

113. Your _____ _____ is determined by the combined forces of the sympathetic and parasympathetic nervous system.

114. According to some physiologists, meditation leads to _____ sympathetic activity and changes opposite to those of the fight-or-flight response.

115. _____ is a malignant tumor of the sympathetic nervous system.

▷ *If you have had difficulty with this section, review pages 297-300.*

UNSCRAMBLE THE WORDS

116. **RONNESU**

117. **APSYENS**

118. **CIATUNOMO**

119. **SHTOMO ULMSEC**

Take the circled letters, unscramble them, and fill in the statement.

What the man hoped the IRS agent would be during his audit.

120.

APPLYING WHAT YOU KNOW

121. Mr. Hemstreet suffered a cerebrovascular accident, and it was determined that the damage affected the left side of his cerebrum. On which side of his body will he most likely notice any paralysis?

122. Baby Dania was born with an excessive accumulation of cerebrospinal fluid in the ventricles. A catheter was placed in the ventricle and the fluid was drained by means of a shunt into the circulatory bloodstream. What condition does this medical history describe?

123. Mrs. Muhlenkamp looked out her window to see a man trapped under the wheel of a car. Although slightly built, Mrs. Muhlenkamp rushed to the car, lifted it, and saved the man. What division of the autonomic nervous system made this seemingly impossible task possible?

124. Lynn's heart raced and her palms became clammy as she watched the monster at the local theater. When the movie was over, however, she told her friends that she was not afraid at all. She appeared to be as calm as before the movie. What division of the autonomic nervous system made this possible?

125. Bill is going to his boss for his annual evaluation. He is planning to ask for a raise and hopes the evaluation will be good. Which subdivision of the autonomic nervous system will be active during this conference? Should he have a large meal before his appointment? Support your answer with facts from the chapter.

126. Word Find

Can you find the 14 terms from the chapter that are listed below? Words may be spelled top to bottom, bottom to top, right to left, left to right, or diagonally.

```
M  C  C  D  Q  S  Y  N  A  P  S  E  Q  G  O
E  N  A  Q  D  W  H  N  W  E  J  N  A  L  W
S  R  O  T  P  E  C  E  R  Y  Z  N  I  S  M
I  D  S  X  E  K  N  O  K  X  G  G  C  Y  Y
J  O  T  R  A  C  T  D  F  L  O  N  E  N  A
R  P  W  E  K  O  H  X  I  D  A  L  H  A  M
F  A  L  O  N  A  Y  O  E  I  I  I  X  P  C
C  M  Z  I  F  D  N  N  L  N  G  Z  U  T  Z
S  I  N  V  C  G  D  G  Z  A  N  A  K  I  P
G  N  A  T  Z  R  O  W  V  A  M  Y  T  C  O
K  E  N  D  O  R  P  H  I  N  S  I  L  C  X
C  P  Q  G  C  J  X  F  J  D  Q  S  N  L  F
X  U  L  I  H  I  G  Q  A  N  S  W  O  E  U
A  I  M  H  Q  E  X  K  D  B  W  Y  T  F  S
A  A  D  A  X  O  C  K  G  B  F  H  B  T  K
```

Axon	Glia	Serotonin
Catecholamines	Microglia	Synapse
Dopamine	Myelin	Synaptic cleft
Endorphins	Oligodendroglia	Tract
Ganglion	Receptors	

DID YOU KNOW?

Although all pain is felt and interpreted in the brain, the brain itself has no pain sensation—even when cut!

THE NERVOUS SYSTEM

Fill in the crossword puzzle.

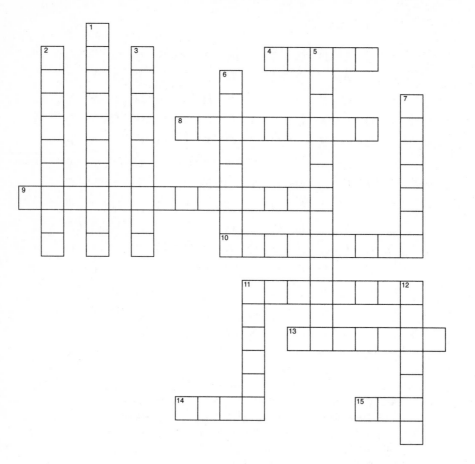

ACROSS

4. Bundle of axons located within the CNS
8. Transmits impulses toward the cell body
9. Neurons that conduct impulses from a ganglion
10. Astrocytes
11. Pia mater
13. Nerve cells
14. Transmits impulses away from the cell body
15. Peripheral nervous system (abbreviation)

DOWN

1. Neuroglia
2. Peripheral beginning of a sensory neuron's dendrite
3. Two-neuron arc (two words)
5. Neurotransmitter
6. Cluster of nerve cell bodies outside the central nervous system
7. Area of brain stem
11. Fatty substance found around some nerve fibers
12. Where impulses are transmitted from one neuron to another

CHECK YOUR KNOWLEDGE

Multiple Choice

Circle the correct answer.

1. What are the neurons called that pick up sensations from receptors and carry them into the brain or spinal cord?
    A. Motor neurons
    B. Central neurons
    C. Interneurons
    D. Sensory neurons

2. What are the brain cavities called that are filled with cerebrospinal fluid?
    A. Hydrocephalics
    B. Ventricles
    C. Mater
    D. Meninges

3. What is the innermost layer of connective tissue that surrounds the brain and spinal cord?
    A. Pia mater
    B. Dura mater
    C. Arachnoid mater
    D. Pons mater

4. A nurse is caring for a patient with a tumor of the cerebellum. In view of the functions of this part of the brain, which of the following symptoms should the nurse expect to observe?
    A. Irregular heartbeat and increased blood pressure
    B. Inability to coordinate body movements
    C. Loss of speech
    D. Inability to control emotions

5. What occurs as a result of stimulation of the sympathetic nervous system?
    A. Accelerated heart rate
    B. Constriction of blood vessels in skeletal muscles
    C. Increased peristalsis
    D. All of the above

6. The autonomic neurotransmitter called *acetylcholine* is released by the:
    A. Sympathetic preganglionic axon
    B. Parasympathetic preganglionic axon
    C. Parasympathetic postganglionic axon
    D. All of the above

7. Which of the following statements about Schwann cells is true?
    A. They are found in the PNS.
    B. They produce myelin.
    C. They are separated by nodes of Ranvier.
    D. All of the above are true.

8. What are areas of the neuron called that secrete neurotransmitters?
    A. Synapses
    B. Synaptic clefts
    C. Synaptic knobs
    D. Gliomas

9. Which of the following statements about the neural tissues called *tracts* is true?
    A. They are located outside of the central nervous system.
    B. They appear gray.
    C. When carrying messages upward they are called *ascending*, and when carrying messages downward they are called *descending*.
    D. All of the above are true.

10. Which of the following statements about the autonomic division of the nervous system is true?
    A. It is composed of two divisions: the sympathetic and parasympathetic.
    B. Autonomic neurotransmitters assist the system in its effort to elicit responses.
    C. The system regulates the body's involuntary functions.
    D. All of the above are true.

Matching

Select the most correct answer from column B for each statement in column A. (Only one answer is correct.)

	Column A		Column B
_____ 11.	Tract	A.	Transmits away from the cell body
_____ 12.	Axon	B.	Interneuron
_____ 13.	Brain stem	C.	White matter
_____ 14.	Neurotransmitter	D.	Cranial nerve
_____ 15.	Reflex arc	E.	Thalamus
_____ 16.	Skin map	F.	Glioma
_____ 17.	Brain tumor	G.	Parkinson's disease
_____ 18.	Diencephalon	H.	Acetylcholine
_____ 19.	Vagus	I.	Dermatome
_____ 20.	"Shaking palsy"	J.	Medulla oblongata

NEURON

1. _____

2. _____

3. _____

4. _____

5. _____

6. _____

7. _____

CRANIAL NERVES

1. _____   7. _____

2. _____   8. _____

3. _____   9. _____

4. _____   10. _____

5. _____   11. _____

6. _____   12. _____

SAGITTAL SECTION OF THE CENTRAL NERVOUS SYSTEM

1. _____   8. _____

2. _____   9. _____

3. _____   10. _____

4. _____   11. _____

5. _____   12. _____

6. _____   13. _____

7. _____

THE CEREBRUM

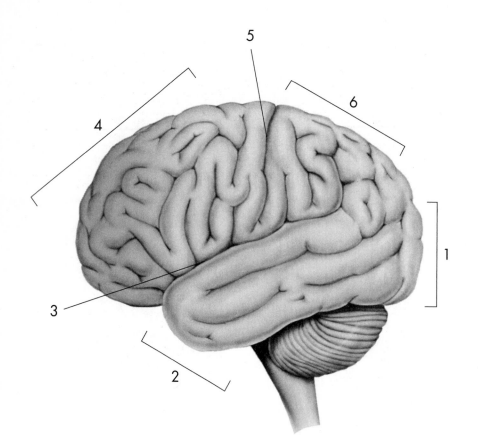

1. _____   4. _____

2. _____   5. _____

3. _____   6. _____

NEURON PATHWAYS

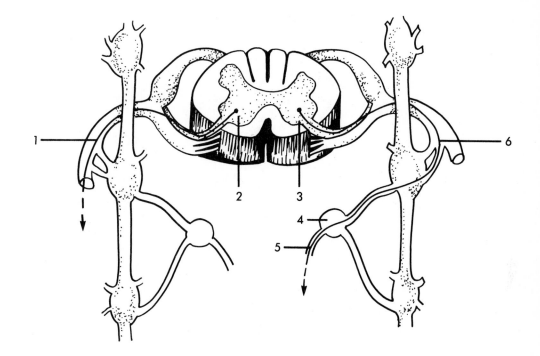

1. _____   4. _____

2. _____   5. _____

3. _____   6. _____

CHAPTER 10

The Senses

Consider this scene for a moment. You are walking along a beautiful beach watching the sunset. You notice the various hues and are amazed at the multitude of shades that cover the sky. The waves are melodious as they splash along the shore and you wiggle your feet with delight as you sense the warm, soft sand trickling between your toes. You sip on a soda and then inhale the fresh salt air as you continue your stroll along the shore. It is a memorable scene, but one that would not be possible without the assistance of your sense organs. The sense organs pick up messages that are sent over nerve pathways to specialized areas in the brain for interpretation. They make communication with and enjoyment of the environment possible. The visual, auditory, tactile, olfactory, and gustatory sense organs not only protect us from danger but also add an important dimension to our daily pleasures of life.

Your study of this chapter will give you an understanding of another one of the systems necessary for homeostasis and survival.

TOPICS FOR REVIEW

Before progressing to Chapter 11, you should review the classification of sense organs and the process for converting a stimulus into a sensation. Your study should also include an understanding of the special sense organs and the general sense organs.

CLASSIFICATION OF SENSE ORGANS
CONVERTING A STIMULUS INTO A SENSATION
GENERAL SENSE ORGANS

Match the term on the left with the proper selection on the right.

_____ 1. Special sense organ   A. Olfactory cells

_____ 2. General sense organ   B. Detects stimuli such as pain or touch

_____ 3. Nose   C. Gustatory cells

_____ 4. Krause's end-bulbs   D. Eye

_____ 5. Taste   E. Touch and possibly cold

▷ *If you have had difficulty with this section, review pages 310-315 and Table 10-1.*

SPECIAL SENSE ORGANS

Eye

Circle the correct answer.

6. The "white" of the eye is more commonly called the:
    A. Choroid
    B. Cornea
    C. Sclera
    D. Retina
    E. None of the above is correct.

7. The "colored" part of the eye is known as the:
    A. Retina
    B. Cornea
    C. Pupil
    D. Sclera
    E. Iris

8. The transparent portion of the sclera, referred to as the "window" of the eye, is the:
    A. Retina
    B. Cornea
    C. Pupil
    D. Iris

9. The mucous membrane that covers the front of the eye is called the:
    A. Cornea
    B. Choroid
    C. Conjunctiva
    D. Ciliary body
    E. None of the above is correct.

10. The structure that can contract or dilate to allow more or less light to enter the eye is the:
    A. Lens
    B. Choroid
    C. Retina
    D. Cornea
    E. Iris

11. When the eye is looking at objects far in the distance, the lens is _____ and the ciliary muscle is _____.
    A. Rounded, contracted
    B. Rounded, relaxed
    C. Slightly rounded, contracted
    D. Slightly curved, relaxed
    E. None of the above is correct

12. The lens of the eye is held in place by the:
    A. Ciliary muscle
    B. Aqueous humor
    C. Vitreous humor
    D. Cornea

13. When the lens loses its elasticity and can no longer bring near objects into focus, the condition is known as:
    A. Glaucoma
    B. Presbyopia
    C. Astigmatism
    D. Strabismus

14. The fluid in front of the lens that is constantly being formed, drained, and replaced in the anterior cavity is the:
    A. Vitreous humor
    B. Protoplasm
    C. Aqueous humor
    D. Conjunctiva

15. If drainage of the aqueous humor is blocked, the internal pressure within the eye will increase and a condition known as _____ could occur.
    A. Presbyopia
    B. Glaucoma
    C. Color blindness
    D. Cataracts

16. The rods and cones are the visual receptors and are located on the:
    A. Sclera
    B. Cornea
    C. Choroid
    D. Retina

17. Photoreception is the sense of:
    A. Vision
    B. Smell
    C. Taste
    D. Balance

18. The "blind spot" may also be referred to as the:
    A. Fovea centralis
    B. Macula lutea
    C. Retinal artery
    D. Optic disc

 If you have had difficulty with this section, review pages 315-318 and Table 10-2.

Visual Disorders

Select the best answer from the choices given and insert the letter in the answer blank.

A. Strabismus   F. Conjunctivitis
B. Retinopathy   G. Nyctalopia
C. Myopia   H. Hyperopia
D. Glaucoma   I. Scotoma
E. Astigmatism   J. Cataracts

_____ 19. Nearsightedness

_____ 20. An irregularity in the cornea

_____ 21. "Pink-eye"

_____ 22. "Cross-eye"

_____ 23. Cloudy spots in the eye's lens

_____ 24. Often caused by diabetes mellitus

_____ 25. Farsightedness

_____ 26. "Night blindness"

_____ 27. Loss of only the center of the visual field

_____ 28. Excessive intraocular pressure caused by abnormal accumulation of aqueous humor

▷ *If you have had difficulty with this section, review pages 318-326.*

Ear

Select the best answer from the choices given and insert the letter in the answer blank.

A. External ear   B. Middle ear   C. Inner ear

_____ 29. Malleus

_____ 30. Perilymph

_____ 31. Incus

_____ 32. Ceruminous glands

_____ 33. Cochlea

_____ 34. Auditory canal

_____ 35. Semicircular canals

_____ 36. Stapes

_____ 37. Tympanic membrane

_____ 38. Organ of Corti

Fill in the blanks.

39. The external ear has two parts: the _____ and the _____ _____ _____.

40. Another name for the tympanic membrane is the _____.

41. The bones of the middle ear are collectively referred to as _____.

42. The stapes presses against a membrane that covers a small opening called the _____ _____.

43. A middle ear infection is called _____ _____.

44. The _____ is located adjacent to the oval window between the semicircular canals and the cochlea.

45. Located within the semicircular canals and the vestibule are _____ for balance and equilibrium.

46. The sensory cells in the _____ _____ are stimulated when movement of the head causes the endolymph to move.

▶ *If you have had difficulty with this section, review pages 326-331.*

Hearing Disorders

Select the best answer from the choices given and insert the letter in the answer blank.

A. Tinnitus
B. Presbycusis
C. Otosclerosis
D. Otitis media
E. Mastoiditis
F. Ménière's disease

_____ 47. Inherited bone disorder that impairs conduction by causing structural irregularities in the stapes

_____ 48. "Ringing in the ear"

_____ 49. Middle ear infection

_____ 50. Untreated otitis media can lead to this condition

_____ 51. Progressive hearing loss associated with aging

_____ 52. Chronic inner ear disease characterized by progressive nerve deafness and vertigo

▶ *If you had difficulty with this section, review pages 331-332.*

TASTE RECEPTORS
SMELL RECEPTORS
GENERAL SENSE ORGANS

Circle the correct answer.

53. Structures known as (papillae or olfactory cells) are found on the tongue.

54. Nerve impulses generated by stimulation of taste buds travel primarily through two (cranial or spinal) nerves.

55. To be detected by olfactory receptors, chemicals must be dissolved in the watery (mucus or plasma) that lines the nasal cavity.

56. The pathways taken by olfactory nerve impulses and the areas where these impulses are interpreted are closely associated with areas of the brain important in (hearing or memory).

57. Receptors responsible for the sense of smell are known as (chemoreceptors or mechanoreceptors).

If you have had difficulty with this section, review pages 332-335.

UNSCRAMBLE THE WORDS

58. **C A L R I E U**

59. **R A E C L S**

60. **L A P I L A E P**

61. **C T V N U C N O I A J**

Take the circled letters, unscramble them, and fill in the statement.

What Mr. Tuttle liked best about his classroom.

62.

APPLYING WHAT YOU KNOW

63. Mr. Nay was an avid swimmer and competed regularly in his age group. He had to withdraw from the last competition due to an infection of his ear. Antibiotics and analgesics were prescribed by the doctor. What is the medical term for his condition?

64. Mrs. Metheny loved the out-of-doors and spent a great deal of her spare time basking in the sun on the beach. Her physician suggested that she begin wearing sunglasses regularly when he noticed milky spots beginning to appear on Mrs. Metheny's lenses. What condition was Mrs. Metheny's physician trying to prevent from occurring?

65. Amanda repeatedly became ill with throat infections during her first few years of school. Lately, however, she has noticed that whenever she has a throat infection, her ears become very sore also. What might be the cause of this additional problem?

66. Richard was hit in the nose with a baseball during practice. His sense of smell was temporarily gone. What nerve receptors were damaged during the injury?

67.　Word Find

Can you find the 19 terms from this chapter that are listed below? Words may be spelled top to bottom, bottom to top, right to left, left to right, or diagonally.

```
M  E  C  H  A  N  O  R  E  C  E  P  T  O  R
H  R  A  T  B  Q  I  R  T  B  N  H  M  A  E
P  F  T  Y  R  O  T  C  A  F  L  O  X  R  C
G  U  A  Y  I  N  A  I  H  C  A  T  S  U  E
G  P  R  A  C  E  R  U  M  E  N  O  P  X  P
I  E  A  I  P  O  Y  B  S  E  R  P  K  D  T
W  L  C  P  L  Y  N  E  Y  K  E  I  T  O  O
C  Q  T  O  I  B  R  J  B  S  F  G  L  M  R
Z  U  S  R  C  L  E  O  U  J  R  M  N  N  S
F  D  M  E  O  H  L  Q  T  N  A  E  Y  I  S
H  I  D  P  N  D  L  A  M  A  C  N  X  S  Z
A  M  L  Y  E  S  S  E  E  D  T  T  M  Z  H
D  D  M  H  S  F  E  X  A  Y  I  S  I  I  A
J  C  G  N  J  T  I  S  L  P  O  G  U  V  J
P  H  G  Y  A  K  H  S  U  C  N  I  S  G  A
```

Cataracts	Gustatory	Presbyopia
Cerumen	Hyperopia	Receptors
Cochlea	Incus	Refraction
Cones	Mechanoreceptor	Rods
Conjunctiva	Olfactory	Senses
Eustachian	Papillae	
Eye	Photopigment	

DID YOU KNOW?

Glaucoma is the leading cause of blindness among African Americans.

THE SENSES

Fill in the crossword puzzle.

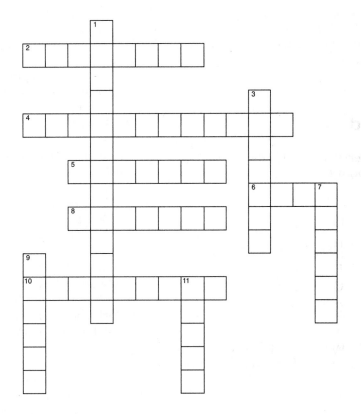

ACROSS

2. Bones of the middle ear
4. Located in anterior cavity in front of lens (two words)
5. External ear
6. Transparent body behind pupil
8. Front part of this coat is the ciliary muscle and iris
10. Membranous labyrinth filled with this fluid

DOWN

1. Located in posterior cavity (two words)
3. Organ of Corti located here
7. White of the eye
9. Innermost layer of the eye
11. Hole in center of the iris

CHECK YOUR KNOWLEDGE

Multiple Choice

Circle the correct answer.

1. Where are the specialized mechanoreceptors of hearing and balance located?
    A. Inner ear
    B. Malleus
    C. Helix
    D. All of the above

2. The organ of Corti is the organ of what sense?
    A. Sight
    B. Hearing
    C. Pressure
    D. Taste

3. Where are taste sensations interpreted?
    A. Cerebral cortex
    B. Area of stimulation
    C. Nasal cavity
    D. None of the above

4. A surgical technique to treat myopia without the use of glasses or contacts is called:
    A. Presbyopia
    B. Removal of cataracts
    C. Radial keratotomy
    D. None of the above

5. Which of the following statements about the cornea is true?
    A. It is a mucous membrane.
    B. It is called the "window of the eye."
    C. It lies behind the iris.
    D. All of the above are true.

6. Which of the following are general sense organs?
    A. Gustatory receptors
    B. Pacinian corpuscles
    C. Olfactory receptors
    D. All of the above

7. The retina contains microscopic receptor cells called:
    A. Mechanoreceptors
    B. Chemoreceptors
    C. Olfactory receptors
    D. Rods and cones

8. Which two involuntary muscles make up the front part of the eye?
    A. Malleus and incus
    B. Iris and ciliary muscle
    C. Retina and pacinian muscle
    D. Sclera and iris

9. Which of the following statements about gustatory sense organs is true?
    A. They are called *taste buds*.
    B. They are innervated by cranial nerves VII and IX.
    C. They work together with the olfactory senses.
    D. All of the above are true.

10. The external ear consists of the:
    A. Auricle and auditory canal
    B. Labyrinth
    C. Corti and cochlea
    D. None of the above

True/False

If the statement is true, write "T" in the answer blank. If the statement is false, correct the statement by circling the incorrect term and inserting the correct term in the answer blank.

_____ 11. The tympanic membrane separates the middle ear from the external ear.

_____ 12. Glaucoma may result from a blockage of flow of vitreous humor.

_____ 13. With the condition of presbyopia, the eye lens loses its elasticity.

_____ 14. The crista ampullaris is located in the nasal cavity.

_____ 15. Myopia occurs when images are focused in front of the retina rather than on it.

_____ 16. Light enters through the pupil, and the size of the pupil is regulated by the iris.

_____ 17. The retina is the innermost layer of the eye. It contains the structures called *rods*.

_____ 18. A commonly used name for the "white of the eye" is the sclera.

_____ 19. The olfactory receptors are chemical receptors.

_____ 20. The organ of Corti contains mechanoreceptors.

EYE

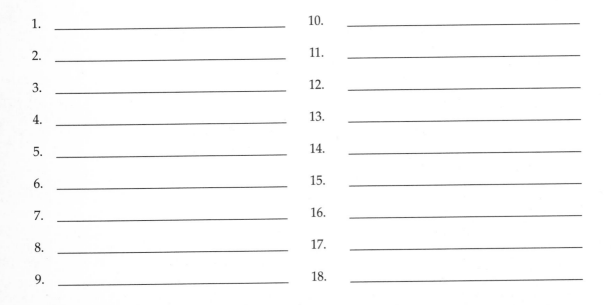

1. _____   10. _____

2. _____   11. _____

3. _____   12. _____

4. _____   13. _____

5. _____   14. _____

6. _____   15. _____

7. _____   16. _____

8. _____   17. _____

9. _____   18. _____

EAR

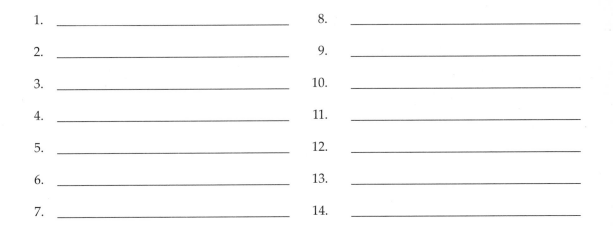

CHAPTER 11

The Endocrine System

The endocrine system has often been compared to a fine concert symphony. When all instruments are playing properly, the sound is melodious. If one instrument plays too loud or too soft, however, it affects the overall quality of the entire performance.

The endocrine system is a ductless system that releases hormones into the bloodstream to help regulate body functions. The pituitary gland may be considered the conductor of the orchestra, because it stimulates many of the endocrine glands to secrete their powerful hormones. All hormones, whether stimulated in this manner or by other control mechanisms, are interdependent. A change in the level of one hormone may affect the level of many other hormones.

In addition to the endocrine glands, prostaglandins, or "tissue hormones," are powerful substances similar to hormones that have been found in a variety of body tissues. These hormones are often produced in a tissue and diffuse only a short distance to act on cells within that area. Prostaglandins influence respiration, blood pressure, gastrointestinal secretions, and the reproductive system and may some day play an important role in the treatment of diseases such as hypertension, asthma, and ulcers.

The endocrine system is a system of communication and control. It differs from the nervous system in that hormones provide a slower, longer-lasting effect than do nerve stimuli and responses. Your understanding of the "system of hormones" will alert you to the mechanism of our emotions, response to stress, growth, chemical balances, and many other body functions.

TOPICS FOR REVIEW

Before progressing to Chapter 12, you should be able to identify and locate the primary endocrine glands of the body. Your understanding should include the hormones that are produced by these glands and the method by which these secretions are regulated. Your study will conclude with the pathological conditions that result from the malfunctioning of this system.

MECHANISMS OF HORMONE ACTION
REGULATION OF HORMONE SECRETION
MECHANISMS OF ENDOCRINE DISEASE
PROSTAGLANDINS

Match the term on the left with the proper selection on the right.

Group A

_____ 1. Pituitary
_____ 2. Parathyroids
_____ 3. Adrenals
_____ 4. Ovaries
_____ 5. Thymus

A. Pelvic cavity
B. Mediastinum
C. Neck
D. Cranial cavity
E. Abdominal cavity

Group B

_____ 6. Negative feedback
_____ 7. Tissue hormones
_____ 8. Second messenger hypothesis
_____ 9. Exocrine glands
_____ 10. Target organ cells

A. Explanation for hormone organ recognition
B. Respond to a particular hormone
C. Prostaglandins
D. Discharge secretions into ducts
E. Specialized homeostatic mechanism that regulates release of hormones

Fill in the blanks.

Nonsteroid hormones work according to the (11) _____

_____ mechanism. According to this concept, a

(12) _____ hormone acts as a (13) _____

_____, providing communication between endocrine glands and

(14) _____ _____. A second messenger,

such as (15) _____ _____, provides com-

munication within a hormone's (16) _____

_____. (17) _____

_____ disrupts the normal negative feedback control of hormones through-

out the body, and may result in tissue damage, sterility, mental imbalance, and a host of life-threatening meta-

bolic problems.

 If you have had difficulty with this section, review pages 342-352.

PITUITARY GLAND
HYPOTHALAMUS

Circle the correct answer.

18. The pituitary gland lies in the _____ bone.
    A. Ethmoid
    B. Sphenoid
    C. Temporal
    D. Frontal
    E. Occipital

19. Which one of the following structures would *not* be stimulated by a tropic hormone from the anterior pituitary?
    A. Ovaries
    B. Testes
    C. Thyroid
    D. Adrenals
    E. Uterus

20. Which one of the following is *not* a function of FSH?
    A. Stimulates the growth of follicles
    B. Stimulates the production of estrogens
    C. Stimulates the growth of seminiferous tubules
    D. Stimulates the interstitial cells of the testes

21. Which one of the following is *not* a function of LH?
    A. Stimulates maturation of a developing follicle
    B. Stimulates the production of estrogens
    C. Stimulates the formation of a corpus luteum
    D. Stimulates sperm cells to mature in the male
    E. Causes ovulation to occur

22. Which one of the following is *not* a function of GH?
    A. Increases glucose catabolism
    B. Increases fat catabolism
    C. Speeds up the movement of amino acids into cells from the bloodstream
    D. All of the above are functions of GH

23. Which one of the following hormones is *not* released by the anterior pituitary gland?
    A. ACTH
    B. TSH
    C. ADH
    D. FSH
    E. LH

24. Which one of the following is *not* a function of prolactin?
    A. Stimulates breast development during pregnancy
    B. Stimulates milk secretion after delivery
    C. Causes the release of milk from glandular cells of the breast
    D. All of the above are functions of prolactin

25. The anterior pituitary gland:
    A. Secretes eight major hormones
    B. Secretes tropic hormones that stimulate other endocrine glands to grow and secrete
    C. Secretes ADH
    D. Secretes oxytocin

26. TSH acts on the:
    A. Thyroid
    B. Thymus
    C. Pineal gland
    D. Testes

27. ACTH stimulates the:
    A. Adrenal cortex
    B. Adrenal medulla
    C. Hypothalamus
    D. Ovaries

28. Which hormone is secreted by the posterior pituitary gland?
    A. MSH
    B. LH
    C. GH
    D. ADH

29. ADH serves the body by:
    A. Initiating labor
    B. Accelerating water reabsorption from urine into the blood
    C. Stimulating the pineal gland
    D. Regulating the calcium/phosphorus levels in the blood

30. The disease caused by hyposecretion of ADH is:
    A. Diabetes insipidus
    B. Diabetes mellitus
    C. Acromegaly
    D. Myxedema

31. The actual production of ADH and oxytocin takes place in which area?
    A. Anterior pituitary
    B. Posterior pituitary
    C. Hypothalamus
    D. Pineal gland

32. Inhibiting hormones are produced by the:
    A. Anterior pituitary
    B. Posterior pituitary
    C. Hypothalamus
    D. Pineal gland

Select the best answer from the choices given and insert the letter in the answer blank.

A. Anterior pituitary   B. Posterior pituitary   C. Hypothalamus

_____ 33. Adenohypophysis

_____ 34. Neurohypophysis

_____ 35. Induced labor

_____ 36. Appetite

_____ 37. Acromegaly

_____ 38. Body temperature

_____ 39. Sex hormones

_____ 40. Tropic hormones

_____ 41. Gigantism

_____ 42. Releasing hormones

▷ *If you have had difficulty with this section, review pages 352-355.*

THYROID GLAND
PARATHYROID GLANDS

Circle the correct answer.

43. The thyroid gland lies (above or below) the larynx.

44. The thyroid gland secretes (calcitonin or glucagon).

45. For thyroxine to be produced in adequate amounts, the diet must contain sufficient (calcium or iodine).

46. Most endocrine glands (do or do not) store their hormones.

47. Colloid is a storage medium for the (thyroid or parathyroid) hormone.

48. Calcitonin (increases or decreases) the concentration of calcium in the blood.

49. Simple goiter results from (hyperthyroidism or hypothyroidism).

50. Hyposecretion of thyroid hormones during the formative years leads to (cretinism or myxedema).

51. The parathyroid glands secrete the hormone (PTH or PTA).

52. Parathyroid hormone tends to (increase or decrease) the concentration of calcium in the blood.

▷ *If you have had difficulty with this section, review pages 355-358.*

ADRENAL GLANDS

Fill in the blanks.

53. The adrenal gland is actually two separate endocrine glands, the _____ _____ and the _____ _____.

54. Hormones secreted by the adrenal cortex are known as _____.

55. The outer zone of the adrenal cortex, the zona glomerulosa, secretes _____.

56. The middle zone, the zona fasciculata, secretes _____.

57. The innermost zone, the zona reticularis, secretes _____ _____.

58. Glucocorticoids act in several ways to increase _____.

59. Glucocorticoids also play an essential part in maintaining _____ _____.

60. The adrenal medulla secretes the hormones _____ and _____.

61. The adrenal medulla may help the body resist _____.

62. A _____ tumor of the adrenal cortex causes masculinizing symptoms to appear in a woman.

Select the best response from the choices given and insert the letter in the answer blank.

A. Adrenal cortex   B. Adrenal medulla

_____ 63. Addison's disease

_____ 64. Anti-immunity

_____ 65. Adrenaline

_____ 66. Cushing's syndrome

_____ 67. Fight-or-flight syndrome

_____ 68. Aldosterone

_____ 69. Androgens

▶ *If you have had difficulty with this section, review pages 358-363.*

PANCREATIC ISLETS
SEX GLANDS
THYMUS
PLACENTA
PINEAL GLAND

Circle the term that does not belong.

70. Alpha cells	Glucagon	Beta cells	Glycogenolysis
71. Insulin	Glucagon	Beta cells	Diabetes mellitus
72. Estrogens	Progesterone	Corpus luteum	Thymosin
73. Chorion	Interstitial cells	Testosterone	Semen
74. Immune system	Mediastinum	Aldosterone	Thymosin
75. Pregnancy	ACTH	Estrogen	Chorion
76. Melatonin	Menstruation	"Third eye"	Semen

Match the term on the left with the proper selection on the right.

Group A

_____ 77. Alpha cells   A. Estrogen
_____ 78. Beta cells   B. Progesterone
_____ 79. Corpus luteum   C. Insulin
_____ 80. Interstitial cells   D. Testosterone
_____ 81. Ovarian follicles   E. Glucagon

Group B

_____ 82. Placenta   A. Melatonin
_____ 83. Pineal gland   B. ANH
_____ 84. Heart atria   C. Testosterone
_____ 85. Testes   D. Thymosin
_____ 86. Thymus   E. Chorionic gonadotropin

▷ *If you have had difficulty with this section, review pages 363-369.*

UNSCRAMBLE THE WORDS

87. **R O O D I I T S C C**

[| | | | | | | | | (○)]

88. **S I U I S E R D**

[| | | (○)(○) | |]

89. **U O O O T D C S I I L R C C G**

[| | | | | | | (○) | | | | |]

90. **R I O D S T E S**

[(○) | | (○) | | |]

Take the circled letters, unscramble them, and fill in the statement.

Why Billy didn't like to take exams.

91. [| | | | |]

APPLYING WHAT YOU KNOW

92. Mrs. Fortner made a routine visit to her physician last week. When the laboratory results came back, the report indicated a high level of chorionic gonadotropin in her urine. What did this mean to Mrs. Fortner?

93. Mrs. Wilcox noticed that her daughter was beginning to take on the secondary sex characteristics of a male. The pediatrician diagnosed the condition as a tumor of an endocrine gland. Where specifically was the tumor located?

94. Mrs. Liddy was pregnant and was 2 weeks past her due date. Her doctor suggested that she enter the hospital and he would induce labor. What hormone will he give Mrs. Liddy?

95. Word Find

Can you find the 16 terms from the chapter that are listed below? Words may be spelled top to bottom, bottom to top, right to left, left to right, or diagonally.

```
S  S  I  S  E  R  U  I  D  M  E  S  I  T  W
N  D  N  X  E  B  A  M  E  D  E  X  Y  M  I
I  I  G  O  N  R  S  G  X  T  I  I  Y  V  B
D  O  M  S  I  N  I  T  E  R  C  C  U  Q  D
N  C  X  S  R  T  N  B  O  T  V  M  Y  O  M
A  I  M  E  C  L  A  C  R  E  P  Y  H  I  X
L  T  Y  R  O  I  E  Z  Q  R  T  J  V  K  F
G  R  E  T  D  P  S  N  I  L  D  J  M  X  N
A  O  O  S  N  I  D  K  I  N  K  S  P  P  O
T  C  P  R  E  T  I  O  G  R  I  F  M  X  G
S  L  M  H  Y  P  O  G  L  Y  C  E  M  I  A
O  A  J  L  H  O  R  M  O  N  E  O  T  G  C
R  C  E  L  T  S  E  L  C  N  P  N  X  U  U
P  I  O  S  W  R  T  X  C  G  U  L  O  E  L
G  G  V  Y  H  M  S  H  Y  K  A  K  N  Q  G
```

Corticoids	Glucagon	Myxedema
Cretinism	Goiter	Prostaglandins
Diabetes	Hormone	Steroids
Diuresis	Hypercalcemia	Stress
Endocrine	Hypoglycemia	
Exocrine	Luteinization	

DID YOU KNOW?

The total daily output of the pituitary gland is less than 1/1,000,000 of a gram, yet this small amount is responsible for stimulating the majority of all endocrine functions.

THE ENDOCRINE SYSTEM

Fill in the crossword puzzle.

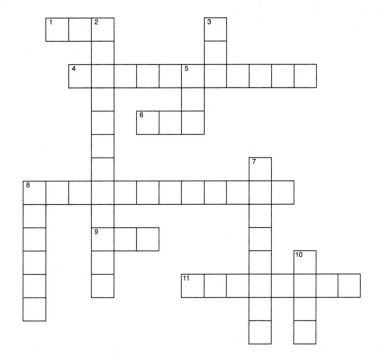

ACROSS

1. Secreted by cells in the walls of the heart's atria
4. Adrenal medulla
6. Estrogens
8. Converts amino acids to glucose
9. Melanin
11. Labor

DOWN

2. Hypersecretion of insulin
3. Antagonist to diuresis
5. Increases calcium concentration
7. Hyposecretion of islets of Langerhans (one word)
8. Hyposecretion of thyroid
10. Adrenal cortex

CHECK YOUR KNOWLEDGE

Multiple Choice

Circle the correct answer.

1. What does the outer zone of the adrenal cortex secrete?
   A. Mineralocorticoids
   B. Sex hormones
   C. Glucocorticoids
   D. Epinephrine

2. From what condition does diabetes insipidus result?
   A. Low insulin levels
   B. High glucagon levels
   C. Low antidiuretic hormone levels
   D. High steroid levels

3. Which of the following statements is true regarding a young child whose growth is stunted, metabolism is low, sexual development is delayed, and mental development is retarded?
   A. The child suffers from cretinism.
   B. The child has an underactive thyroid.
   C. The child could suffer from a pituitary disorder.
   D. All of the above are true.

4. What can result when too much growth hormone is produced by the pituitary gland?
   A. Hyperglycemia
   B. A pituitary giant
   C. Both A and B
   D. None of the above

5. Which of the following glands is *not* regulated by the pituitary?
   A. Thyroid
   B. Ovaries
   C. Adrenals
   D. Thymus

6. Which of the following statements about the antidiuretic hormone is true?
   A. It is released by the posterior lobe of the pituitary.
   B. It causes diabetes insipidus when produced in insufficient amounts.
   C. It decreases urine volume.
   D. All of the above are true.

7. What controls the development of the body's immune system?
   A. Pituitary
   B. Thymus
   C. Pineal body
   D. Thyroid

8. Administration of what would best treat a person suffering from severe allergies?
   A. Gonadocorticoids
   B. Glucagon
   C. Mineralocorticoids
   D. Glucocorticoids

9. What endocrine gland is composed of cell clusters called the *islets of Langerhans*?
   A. Adrenals
   B. Thyroid
   C. Pituitary
   D. Pancreas

10. Which of the following statements concerning prostaglandins is true?
    A. They control activities of widely separated organs.
    B. They can be called *tissue hormones.*
    C. They diffuse over long distances to act on cells.
    D. All of the above are true.

Matching

Select the most correct answer from column B for each item in column A. (Only one answer is correct.)

Column A

_____ 11. Goiter
_____ 12. Ovulation
_____ 13. Diabetes mellitus
_____ 14. Lactation
_____ 15. Diabetes insipidus
_____ 16. Chorionic gonadotropins
_____ 17. Cushing's syndrome
_____ 18. Labor
_____ 19. Acromegaly
_____ 20. Hypercalcemia

Column B

A. Glucocorticoid hormones
B. Antidiuretic hormone
C. Calcitonin
D. Oxytocin
E. Growth hormone
F. Placenta
G. Luteinizing hormone
H. Insulin
I. Prolactin
J. Thyroid hormones

ENDOCRINE GLANDS

1. _____

2. _____

3. _____

4. _____

5. _____

6. _____

7. _____

8. _____

9. _____

10. _____

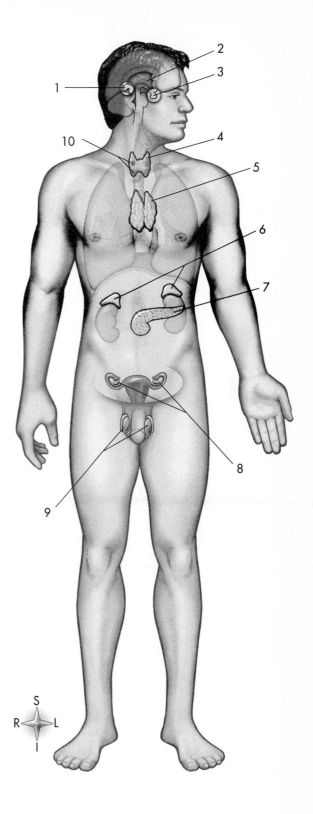

CHAPTER 12

Blood

Blood, the river of life, is the body's primary means of transportation. Although it is the respiratory system that provides oxygen for the body, the digestive system that provides nutrients, and the urinary system that eliminates wastes, none of these functions could be provided for the individual cells without the blood. In less than 1 minute, a drop of blood will complete a trip through the entire body, distributing nutrients and collecting the wastes of metabolism.

Blood is divided into plasma (the liquid portion of blood) and the formed elements (the blood cells). There are three types of blood cells: red blood cells, white blood cells, and platelets. Together these cells and plasma provide a means of transportation that delivers the body's daily necessities.

Although all of us have red blood cells that are similar in shape, we have different blood types. Blood types are identified by the presence of certain antigens in the red blood cells. Every person's blood belongs to one of four main blood groups: Type A, B, AB, or O. Any one of the four groups or "types" may or may not have the Rh factor present in the red blood cells. If an individual has a specific antigen called the Rh factor present in his or her blood, the blood is Rh positive. If this factor is missing, the blood is Rh negative. Approximately, 85% of the population has the Rh factor (Rh positive) while 15% do not have the Rh factor (Rh negative).

Your understanding of this chapter will be necessary to prepare a proper foundation for the circulatory system.

TOPICS FOR REVIEW

Before progressing to Chapter 13, you should have an understanding of the structure and function of blood plasma and cells. Your review should also include an understanding of blood types and Rh factors.

BLOOD COMPOSITION

Circle the correct answer.

1. Which one of the following substances is *not* a part of the plasma?
   A. Water
   B. Proteins
   C. Nutrients
   D. Waste products
   E. Formed elements

2. The normal volume of blood in an adult is approximately:
   A. 2-3 pints
   B. 2-3 quarts
   C. 2-3 gallons
   D. 4-6 liters

3. Blood is normally:
   A. Very acidic
   B. Slightly acidic
   C. Neutral
   D. Slightly alkaline

4. PolyHeme is a/an:
   A. Artificial blood
   B. Antigen
   C. Antibody
   D. Plasma volume expander

▶ *If you have had difficulty with this section, review pages 379-381.*

5. Donated blood:
   A. Must be "typed and cross matched"
   B. Can only be stored for 6 weeks
   C. Is most valuable during the "golden hour"
   D. All of the above

BLOOD TYPES
RH FACTOR

6. Fill in the blank areas.

Blood Type	Antigen Present in RBC	Antibody Present in Plasma
A		Anti-B
B	B	
AB		None
O	None	

Fill in the blanks.

7. An _____ is a substance that can stimulate the body to make antibodies.

8. An _____ is a substance made by the body in response to stimulation by an antigen.

9. Many antibodies react with their antigens to clump or _____ them.

10. If a baby is born to an Rh-negative mother and Rh-positive father, it may develop the disease _____ _____.

11. The term "Rh" is used because the antigen was first discovered in the blood of a _____ _____.

12. The universal donor blood is _____.

13. The universal recipient blood is _____.

▶ *If you have had difficulty with this section, review pages 381-384.*

BLOOD PLASMA AND BLOOD ELEMENTS

Circle the correct answer.

14. Another name for white blood cells is:
    A. Erythrocytes
    B. Leukocytes
    C. Thrombocytes
    D. Platelets

15. Another name for platelets is:
    A. Neutrophils
    B. Eosinophils
    C. Thrombocytes
    D. Erythrocytes

16. Pernicious anemia is caused by:
    A. A lack of vitamin B_{12}
    B. Hemorrhage
    C. Radiation
    D. Bleeding ulcers

17. The laboratory test called *hematocrit* tells the physician the volume of:
    A. White cells in a blood sample
    B. Red cells in a blood sample
    C. Platelets in a blood sample
    D. Plasma in a blood sample

18. An example of a nongranular leukocyte is a/an:
    A. Platelet
    B. Erythrocyte
    C. Eosinophil
    D. Monocyte

19. An excess of red blood cells is known as:
    A. Erythropenia
    B. Erythroplasia
    C. Polycythemia
    D. Anemia

20. A critical component of hemoglobin is:
    A. Potassium
    B. Calcium
    C. Vitamin K
    D. Iron

21. Sickle cell anemia is caused by:
    A. The production of an abnormal type of hemoglobin
    B. The production of excessive neutrophils
    C. The production of excessive platelets
    D. The production of abnormal leukocytes

22. The practice of using blood transfusions to increase oxygen delivery to muscles during athletic events is called:
    A. Blood antigen
    B. Blood doping
    C. Blood agglutination
    D. Blood proofing

23. One of the most useful and frequently performed clinical blood tests is called the:
    A. WBC
    B. CBC
    C. RBC
    D. Hematocrit

24. Which one of the following types of cells is not a granular leukocyte?
    A. Neutrophil
    B. Monocyte
    C. Basophil
    D. Eosinophil

25. If a blood cell has no nucleus and is shaped like a biconcave disc, then the cell most likely is a/an:
    A. Platelet
    B. Lymphocyte
    C. Basophil
    D. Eosinophil
    E. Red blood cell

26. Red bone marrow forms all kinds of blood cells except some:
    A. Platelets and basophils
    B. Lymphocytes and monocytes
    C. Red blood cells
    D. Neutrophils and eosinophils

27. Myeloid tissue is found in all but which one of the following locations?
    A. Sternum
    B. Ribs
    C. Wrist bones
    D. Hip bones
    E. Cranial bones

28. Lymphatic tissue is found in which of the following locations?
    A. Lymph nodes
    B. Thymus
    C. Spleen
    D. All of the above contain lymphatic tissue.

29. The "buffy coat" layer in a hematocrit tube contains:
    A. Red blood cells and platelets
    B. Plasma only
    C. Platelets only
    D. White blood cells and platelets
    E. None of the above is correct

30. The hematocrit value for red blood cells is _____%.
    A. 75
    B. 60
    C. 50
    D. 45
    E. 35

31. An unusually low white blood cell count would be termed:
    A. Leukemia
    B. Leukopenia
    C. Leukocytosis
    D. Anemia
    E. None of the above is correct.

32. Most of the oxygen transported in the blood is carried by:
    A. Platelets
    B. Plasma
    C. White blood cells
    D. Red blood cells
    E. None of the above is correct.

33. The most numerous of the phagocytes are the _____.
    A. Lymphocytes
    B. Neutrophils
    C. Basophils
    D. Eosinophils
    E. Monocytes

34. Which one of the following types of cells is *not* phagocytic?
    A. Neutrophils
    B. Eosinophils
    C. Lymphocytes
    D. Monocytes
    E. All of the above are phagocytic cells.

35. Which of the following cell types functions in the immune process?
    A. Neutrophils
    B. Lymphocytes
    C. Monocytes
    D. Basophils
    E. Reticuloendothelial cells

36. Vitamin K stimulates liver cells to increase the synthesis of:
    A. Prothrombin
    B. Thrombin
    C. Platelets
    D. Heparin
    E. Calcium

37. If part of a clot dislodges and circulates through the bloodstream, the dislodged part is called a/an:
    A. Thrombus
    B. Thrombosis
    C. Anticoagulant
    D. Clotting factor
    E. Embolus

38. This disease usually occurs as a result of the destruction of bone marrow by toxic chemicals or radiation.
    A. Folate-deficiency anemia
    B. Aplastic anemia
    C. Hemolytic anemia
    D. Sickle cell anemia

39. An example of a hemolytic anemia is:
    A. Folate-deficiency anemia
    B. Aplastic anemia
    C. Sickle cell anemia
    D. Pernicious anemia

40. The disease that results from a failure to form blood clotting factor VIII is:
    A. Hemophilia
    B. Thrombocytopenia
    C. Thrombophlebitis
    D. None of the above

41. A special type of white blood cell count used as a diagnostic tool is known as a/an:
    A. Leukopenia
    B. Granulocyte count
    C. Differential WBC count
    D. CBC

▶ *If you have had difficulty with this section, review pages 384-399.*

APPLYING WHAT YOU KNOW

42. Mrs. Florez's blood type is O positive. Her husband's type is O negative. Her newborn baby's blood type is O negative. Is there any need for concern with this combination?

43. After Mrs. Freund's baby was born, the doctor applied a gauze dressing for a short time on the umbilical cord. He also gave the baby a dose of vitamin K. Why did the doctor perform these two procedures?

44. Valerie was a teenager with a picky appetite. She loved junk food and seldom ate properly. She complained of being tired all the time. A visit to her doctor revealed a hemoglobin of 10 and RBCs that are classified as hypochromic. What condition does Valerie have?

45. Word Find

Can you find the 24 terms from this chapter that are listed below? Words may be spelled top to bottom, bottom to top, right to left, left to right, or diagonally.

```
H S H K L S U L O B M E A E S
K E E V M Z H E P A R I N D N
D T M F A C T O R Y E T I Q P
O Y A O H N B A T Q Y A R A R
N C T J G W E H N P N L B U D
O O O S Q L R M E T I S I P M
R K C E M O O N I H I Q F W W
H U R T C N I B P A S G Z T G
E E I Y O B O O I V E W E T X
S L T C M D S E C N R T U N R
U E Y O Y A I M E K U E L Y S
S T R G B S T H R O M B U S Q
E H Z A M S A L P N D Z P O N
T E N H F P D A P M E E I B W
E W B P H K B O N C K W X V J
```

AIDS	Factor	Phagocytes
Anemia	Fibrin	Plasma
Antibody	Hematocrit	Recipient
Antigen	Hemoglobin	Rhesus
Basophil	Heparin	Serum
Donor	Leukemia	Thrombin
Embolus	Leukocytes	Thrombus
Erythrocytes	Monocyte	Type

BLOOD

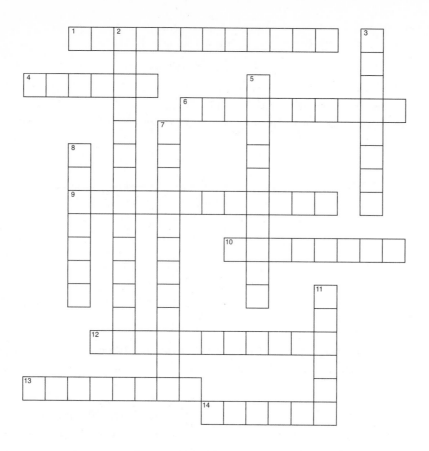

ACROSS

1. Abnormally high WBC count
4. Final stage of clotting process
6. Oxygen-carrying mechanism of blood
9. To engulf and digest microbes
10. Stationary blood clot
12. RBC
13. Circulating blood clot
14. Liquid portion of blood

DOWN

2. Type O (two words)
3. Substances that stimulate the body to make antibodies
5. Type of leukocyte
7. Platelets
8. Prevents clotting of blood
11. Inability of the blood to carry sufficient oxygen

DID YOU KNOW?

Blood products are good for approximately 3 to 6 weeks, but fresh frozen plasma is good for at least 6 months.

CHECK YOUR KNOWLEDGE

Multiple Choice

Circle the correct answer.

1. Which of the following statements is false?
   A. Sickle cell anemia is caused by a genetic defect.
   B. Leukemia is characterized by a low number of WBCs.
   C. Polycythemia is characterized by an abnormally high number of erythrocytes.
   D. Pernicious anemia is caused by a lack of vitamin B_{12}.

2. Deficiency in the number or function of erythrocytes is called:
   A. Leukemia
   B. Anemia
   C. Polycythemia
   D. Leukopenia

3. Which of the following statements does *not* describe a characteristic of leukocytes?
   A. They are disk-shaped cells that do not contain a nucleus.
   B. They have the ability to fight infection.
   C. They provide defense against certain parasites.
   D. They provide immune defense.

4. Which of the following substances is *not* found in serum?
   A. Clotting factors
   B. Water
   C. Hormones
   D. All of the above substances are found in serum.

5. Which of the following substances is *not* found in blood plasma?
   A. Water
   B. Oxygen
   C. Hormones
   D. All of the above substances are found in blood plasma.

6. An allergic reaction may increase the number of:
   A. Eosinophils
   B. Neutrophils
   C. Lymphocytes
   D. Monocytes

7. What is a blood clot that is moving through the body called?
   A. Embolism
   B. Fibrosis
   C. Heparin
   D. Thrombosis

8. When could difficulty with the Rh blood factor arise?
   A. When an Rh-negative man and woman produce a child.
   B. When an Rh-positive man and woman produce a child.
   C. When an Rh-positive woman and an Rh-negative man produce a child.
   D. When an Rh-negative woman and an Rh-positive man produce a child.

9. What is the primary function of hemoglobin?
   A. To fight infection
   B. To make blood clots
   C. To carry oxygen
   D. To transport hormones

10. Are any of the following steps *not* involved in blood clot formation?
    A. A blood vessel is injured and platelet factors are formed.
    B. Thrombin is converted into prothrombin.
    C. Fibrinogen is converted into fibrin.
    D. All of the above are involved in blood clot formation.

Matching

Select the most correct answer from column B for each item in column A. (Only one answer is correct.)

Column A

_____ 11. Lymphocytes
_____ 12. Erythrocytes
_____ 13. Type AB
_____ 14. Basophils
_____ 15. Leukemia
_____ 16. Platelets
_____ 17. Type O
_____ 18. Rh factor
_____ 19. Red bone marrow
_____ 20. Neutrophils

Column B

A. Heparin
B. Contains anti-A and anti-B antibodies
C. Clotting
D. Immunity
E. Erythroblastosis fetalis
F. Anemia
G. Cancer
H. Contains A and B antigens
I. Myeloid tissue
J. Phagocytosis

HUMAN BLOOD CELLS

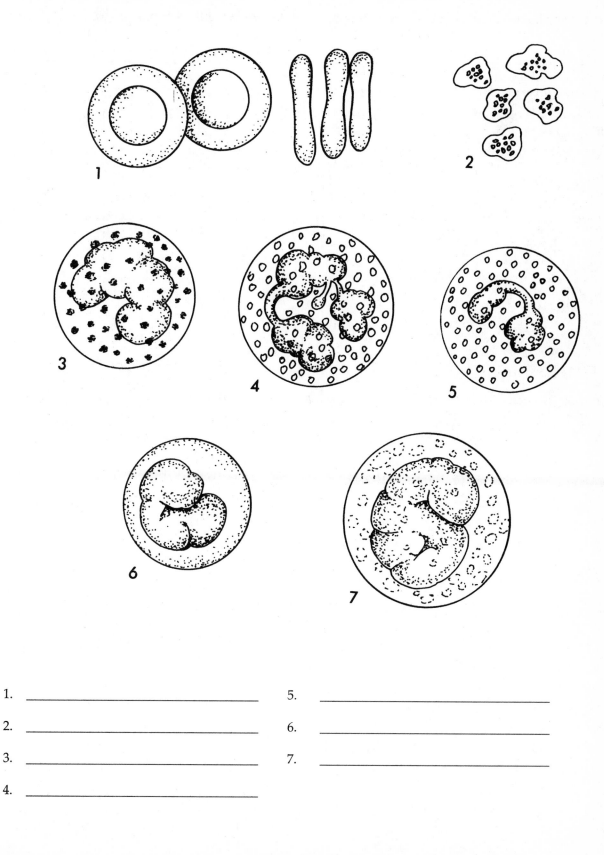

1. _____

2. _____

3. _____

4. _____

5. _____

6. _____

7. _____

BLOOD TYPING

Using the key below, draw the appropriate reaction with the donor's blood in the circles.

Recipient's blood		Reactions with donor's blood			
RBC antigens	Plasma antibodies	Donor type O	Donor type A	Donor type B	Donor type AB
None (Type O)	Anti-A Anti-B	○	○	○	○
A (Type A)	Anti-B	○	○	○	○
B (Type B)	Anti-A	○	○	○	○
AB (Type AB)	(none)	○	○	○	○

Normal blood   Agglutinated blood

CHAPTER 13

The Heart and Heart Disease

The heart is actually two pumps—one moves blood to the lungs, the other pushes it out into the body. These two functions seem rather elementary in comparison to the complex and numerous functions performed by most of the other body organs, and yet if this pump stops, within a few short minutes all life ceases.

The heart is divided into two upper compartments called *atria,* or receiving chambers, and two lower compartments, or discharging chambers, called *ventricles.* By age 45, approximately 300,000 tons of blood will have passed through these chambers to be circulated to the blood vessels. This closed system of circulation provides distribution of blood to the entire body (systemic circulation) and to specific regions, such as the pulmonary circulation or coronary circulation.

The beating of the heart must be coordinated in a rhythmic manner if the heart is to pump effectively. This is achieved by electrical impulses that are stimulated by specialized structures embedded in the walls of the heart. The sinoatrial node, atrioventricular node, bundle of His, and Purkinje fibers combine efforts to produce the tiny electrical currents necessary to contract the heart. Any interruption or failure of this system may result in serious pathology or death.

A healthy heart is necessary to pump sufficient blood throughout the body to nourish and oxygenate cells continuously. Your review of this chapter will provide you with an understanding of this vital organ that is necessary for survival.

TOPICS FOR REVIEW

Before progressing to Chapter 14 you should have an understanding of the structure and function of the heart. Your review should include a study of the coronary circulation and the conduction system of the heart. Your study should conclude with an understanding of the major coronary diseases and disorders.

LOCATION, SIZE, AND POSITION OF THE HEART
ANATOMY OF THE HEART

Fill in the blanks.

1. The system that supplies our cells' transportation needs is the _____
   _____.

2. The _____ or blunt point at the lower edge of the heart lies on the diaphragm, pointing to the left.

3. The _____ _____ divides the heart into right and left sides between the atria.

4. The _____ are the two upper chambers of the heart.

5. The _____ are the two lower chambers of the heart.

6. The cardiac muscle tissue is referred to as the _____.

7. Inflammation of the heart lining is _____.

8. The two AV valves are _____ and
_____.

9. The inner layer of the pericardium is called the _____
_____ or _____.

10. The outer layer of pericardium is called _____
_____.

11. If the pericardium becomes inflamed, a condition called _____ results.

12. The _____ _____ are located between the two ventricular chambers and the large arteries that carry blood away from the heart when contraction occurs.

13. A _____
_____ is a condition caused when the flaps of this valve extend back into the left atrium, causing the valve to leak.

14. _____ _____
_____ is cardiac damage resulting from a delayed inflammatory response to a streptococcal infection that occurs most often in children.

▷ *If you have had difficulty with this section, review pages 410-417.*

HEART SOUNDS
BLOOD FLOW THROUGH THE HEART
CORONARY CIRCULATION AND CORONARY HEART DISEASE
HEART FAILURE

Select the best answer.

_____ 15. Movement of blood from the left ventricle through the body

_____ 16. Blood clot

_____ 17. Myocardial infarction

_____ 18. Abnormal heart sound often caused by disorders of the valves

_____ 19. Movement of blood from the right ventricle to the lungs

_____ 20. Hardening of the arteries

_____ 21. Severe chest pain

_____ 22. High blood pressure

_____ 23. Blood returns to the left atrium through these structures

_____ 24. Treatment for certain coronary disorders

A. Heart murmur

B. Pulmonary circulation

C. Embolism

D. Heart attack

E. Angina pectoris

F. Systemic circulation

G. Atherosclerosis

H. Hypertension

I. Coronary bypass

J. Pulmonary veins

CARDIAC CYCLE
CONDUCTION SYSTEM OF THE HEART

Circle the correct answer.

25. The heart beats at an average rate of _____ beats per minute.
    A. 50
    B. 72
    C. 100
    D. 120

26. Each complete beat of the heart is called:
    A. Cardiac output
    B. Stroke volume
    C. A cardiac cycle
    D. A contraction

27. The pacemaker of the heart is also known as the:
    A. SA node
    B. AV node
    C. AV bundle
    D. Purkinje fibers

28. A rapid heart rhythm, over 100 beats per minutes, is referred to as:
    A. Bradycardia
    B. Sinus arrhythmia
    C. Tachycardia
    D. Premature contractions

29. The term _____ describes the electrical activity that triggers contraction of the heart muscle.
    A. Depolarization
    B. Repolarization
    C. AV node block
    D. Cardiac arrhythmia

30. A diagnostic tool that uses ultrasound to detect valve and heart disorders is known as a/an:
    A. Electrocardiogram
    B. Pacemaker
    C. TPA
    D. Echocardiogram

31. Frequent premature contractions can lead to:
    A. Extra systoles
    B. Bradycardia
    C. Fibrillation
    D. Heart failure

32. A drug that slows and increases the strength of cardiac contractions is:
    A. Digitalis
    B. Nitroglycerin
    C. Calcium-channel blocker
    D. Anticoagulant

33. Congestive heart failure inevitably causes:
    A. Extra systole
    B. Pulmonary edema
    C. Fibrillation
    D. Bradycardia

34. Failure of the right side of the heart due to blockage of pulmonary blood flow is called:
    A. Cardiomyopathy
    B. Ventricular fibrillation
    C. Cor pulmonale
    D. TPA

35. A nonmedical rescuer can defibrillate a victim in ventricular fibrillation with the use of a/an:
    A. AED
    B. Beta-blocker
    C. Demand pacemaker
    D. ECG

36. Coumadin and dicumarol are examples of commonly used oral:
    A. Beta-blockers
    B. Nitroglycerines
    C. Calcium-channel blockers
    D. Anticoagulants

▶ *If you have had difficulty with this section review pages 417-427.*

APPLYING WHAT YOU KNOW

37. Else was experiencing angina pectoris. Her doctor suggested a surgical procedure that would require the removal of a vein from another region of her body. They would then use the vein to bypass a partial blockage in her coronary arteries. What is this procedure called?
38. Mr. Stuckey has a heart block. His electrical impulses are being blocked from reaching the ventricles. An electrical device that causes ventricular contractions at a rate necessary to maintain circulation is being considered as possible treatment for his condition. What is this device?
39. Mrs. Haygood was diagnosed with an acute case of endocarditis. What is the real danger of this diagnosis?
40. Jeanne's homework assignment was to be able to demonstrate knowledge of the flow of blood through the heart. Can you help her?

Trace the blood flow through the heart by numbering the following structures in the correct sequence. Start with number 1 for the vena cava and proceed until you have numbered all 12 structures.

_____ Tricuspid valve   _____ Pulmonary veins

_____ Pulmonary arteries   _____ Pulmonary semilunar valve

_____ Bicuspid valve   _____ Left ventricle

_____ Vena cava   _____ Right atrium

_____ Right ventricle   _____ Left atrium

_____ Aorta   _____ Aortic semilunar valve

41. Word Find

Can you find the 12 terms from this chapter that are listed below? Words may be spelled top to bottom, bottom to top, right to left, left to right, or diagonally.

```
P W S T L W G V F V W Q U S Y
U T X U L Q L V M J W O U J D
R E S P E B S W Z W K N X Q Y
K V Y T E V E N T R I C L E S
I F K U O E L O T S Y S X V R
N G Z O A R G A Y C M X F K H
J B B C U J T R V K P Y P W Y
E V L A V R A N U L I M E S T
F D T I Z N H I Y A A D U T H
I T B D O D S H Y P U R W I M
B P E R I C A R D I U M T D I
E M O A B R A D Y C A R D I A
R C U C E N D O C A R D I U M
S A I D R A C Y H C A T B Y P
```

Bradycardia	Endocardium	Semilunar valve
Cardiac output	Mitral valve	Systole
Coronary sinus	Pericardium	Tachycardia
Dysrhythmia	Purkinje fibers	Ventricle

DID YOU KNOW?

Your heart pumps more than 5 quarts of blood every minute—that's 2,000 gallons a day!

HEART AND HEART DISEASE

Fill in the crossword puzzle.

ACROSS

1. Inflammation of the pericardium
3. A condition in which muscle fibers contract out of step with each other
6. Disease of the myocardial tissue
8. Also known as the *visceral pericardium*
9. Relaxation of the heart
10. Upper chambers of the heart

DOWN

2. Heart specialist
4. Also known as the *sinoatrial node*
5. Complex that occurs as a result of depolarization of the ventricles
7. Also known as the *mitral valve*
8. Graphic record of the heart's electrical activity

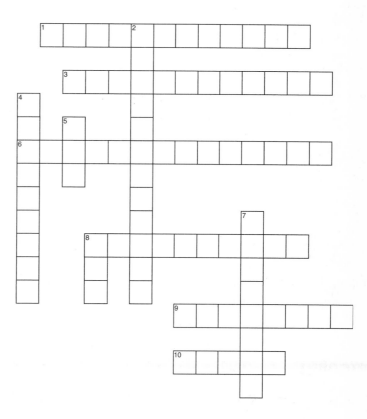

CHECK YOUR KNOWLEDGE

Multiple Choice

Circle the correct answer.

1. The superior vena cava carries blood to the:
   A. Left ventricle
   B. Coronary arteries
   C. Right atrium
   D. Pulmonary veins

2. Which of the following events, if any, does *not* precede ventricular contraction?
   A. P wave
   B. Atrial depolarization
   C. Ventricular depolarization
   D. All of these events precede contraction

3. Which of the following pairs is mismatched?
   A. Angina pectoris—chest pain
   B. Congestive heart failure—left-sided heart failure
   C. Tachycardia—slow heart rhythm
   D. Dysrhythmia—heart block

4. Which of the following statements is *not* true regarding pericarditis?
    A. It may be caused by infection or trauma.
    B. It often causes severe chest pain.
    C. It may result in impairment of the pumping action of the heart.
    D. All of the above statements are true.

5. The outside covering that surrounds and protects the heart is called the:
    A. Endocardium
    B. Myocardium
    C. Pericardium
    D. Ectocardium

6. Thin-walled upper heart cavities that receive blood from veins are called:
    A. Chordae tendineae
    B. Atria
    C. Pericardia
    D. Ventricles

7. A valve that permits blood to flow from the right ventricle into the pulmonary artery is called:
    A. Tricuspid
    B. Mitral
    C. Aortic semilunar
    D. Pulmonary semilunar

8. Ventricular contraction of the heart occurs *immediately after* depolarization of the:
    A. Purkinje fibers
    B. Atrioventricular node
    C. Sinoatrial node
    D. Bundle of His

9. A variation in heart rate during the breathing cycle is called:
    A. Mitral valve prolapse
    B. Fibrillation
    C. Sinus dysrhythmia
    D. None of the above

10. Heart implants:
    A. Allow patients to move around freely without external pumps.
    B. Are artificial hearts that are made of biologically inert synthetic materials.
    C. Weigh approximately 2 pounds.
    D. All of the above are true.

Matching

Select the correct answer from column B for each item in column A. (Only one answer is correct.)

Column A

_____ 11. Heart attack
_____ 12. QRS complex
_____ 13. Systole
_____ 14. Pulmonary circulation
_____ 15. Bicuspid
_____ 16. Heart compression
_____ 17. Heart muscle
_____ 18. Pacemaker
_____ 19. T wave
_____ 20. Chest pain

Column B

A. Sinoatrial node
B. Cardiac tamponade
C. Myocardium
D. Ventricular repolarization
E. Angina pectoris
F. Myocardial infarction
G. Ventricular depolarization
H. Ventricular contraction
I. Lungs
J. Mitral

THE HEART

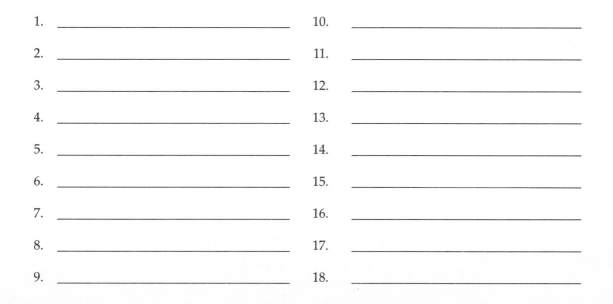

1. _____   10. _____

2. _____   11. _____

3. _____   12. _____

4. _____   13. _____

5. _____   14. _____

6. _____   15. _____

7. _____   16. _____

8. _____   17. _____

9. _____   18. _____

CONDUCTION SYSTEM OF THE HEART

1. _____   8. _____

2. _____   9. _____

3. _____   10. _____

4. _____   11. _____

5. _____   12. _____

6. _____   13. _____

7. _____

NORMAL ECG DEFLECTIONS

1. _____   3. _____

2. _____

CHAPTER 14

The Circulation of the Blood

One hundred thousand miles of blood vessels make up the elaborate transportation system that circulates materials for energy, growth and repair, and eliminates wastes from your body. These vessels, called *arteries, veins,* and *capillaries,* serve different functions. Arteries carry blood from the heart, veins carry blood to the heart, and capillaries are exchange vessels, or connecting links, between the arteries and veins. The pumping action of the heart keeps blood moving through the closed system of vessels. This closed system of circulation provides distribution of blood to the entire body (systemic circulation) and to specific regions such as the pulmonary circulation or hepatic portal circulation.

Blood pressure is the force of blood in the vessels. This force is highest in the arteries and lowest in the veins. Normal blood pressure varies among individuals and depends on the volume of blood in the arteries. The larger the volume of blood in the arteries, the more pressure is exerted on the walls of the arteries, and the higher the arterial pressure. Conversely, the less blood in the arteries, the lower the blood pressure.

A functional cardiovascular system is vital for survival because without circulation, tissues would lack a supply of oxygen and nutrients. Waste products would begin to accumulate and could become toxic. Your review of this system will provide you with an understanding of the complex transportation mechanism of the body necessary for survival.

TOPICS FOR REVIEW

Before progressing to Chapter 15, you should have an understanding of the structure and function of the blood vessels. Your review should include a study of systemic, pulmonary, hepatic portal, and fetal circulation and should conclude with a thorough understanding of blood pressure, pulse, and circulatory shock.

BLOOD VESSELS

Match the term on the left with the proper selection on the right.

_____ 1. Arteries

_____ 2. Veins

_____ 3. Capillaries

_____ 4. Tunica externa

_____ 5. Precapillary sphincters

_____ 6. Superior vena cava

_____ 7. Aorta

A. Smooth muscle cells that guard the entrance to capillaries

B. Carry blood to the heart

C. Carry blood into the venules

D. Carry blood away from the heart

E. Largest vein

F. Largest artery

G. Outermost layer of arteries and veins

▶ *If you have difficulty with this section, review pages 434-441.*

DISORDERS OF BLOOD VESSELS

Match the definition on the left with the proper term on the right.

_____ 8.   Hardening of the arteries

_____ 9.   Decreased blood supply to a tissue

_____ 10. Tissue death

_____ 11. Necrosis that has progressed to decay

_____ 12. A type of arteriosclerosis caused by lipids

_____ 13. A section of an artery that has become abnormally widened

_____ 14. Varicose veins in the rectum

_____ 15. Vein inflammation

_____ 16. Clot formation

_____ 17. Cerebral vascular accident

A. Atherosclerosis

B. Ischemia

C. Aneurysm

D. Necrosis

E. Gangrene

F. Hemorrhoids

G. Phlebitis

H. Stroke

I. Arteriosclerosis

J. Thrombus

▶ *If you have had difficulty with this section, review pages 441-444.*

CIRCULATION OF BLOOD

Circle the correct answer.

18. The aorta carries blood out of the:
    A. Right atrium
    B. Left atrium
    C. Right ventricle
    D. Left ventricle
    E. None of the above

19. The superior vena cava returns blood to the:
    A. Left atrium
    B. Left ventricle
    C. Right atrium
    D. Right ventricle
    E. None of the above

20. The _____ function as exchange vessels.
    A. Venules
    B. Capillaries
    C. Arteries
    D. Arterioles
    E. Veins

21. Blood returns from the lungs during pulmonary circulation via the:
    A. Pulmonary artery
    B. Pulmonary veins
    C. Aorta
    D. Inferior vena cava

22. The hepatic portal circulation serves the body by:
    A. Removing excess glucose and storing it in the liver as glycogen
    B. Detoxifying blood
    C. Assisting the body to maintain proper blood glucose balance
    D. All of the above

23. The structure used to bypass the liver in the fetal circulation is the:
    A. Foramen ovale
    B. Ductus venosus
    C. Ductus arteriosus
    D. Umbilical vein

24. The foramen ovale serves the fetal circulation by:
    A. Connecting the aorta and the pulmonary artery
    B. Shunting blood from the right atrium directly into the left atrium
    C. Bypassing the liver
    D. Bypassing the lungs

25. The structure used to connect the aorta and pulmonary artery in the fetal circulation is the:
    A. Ductus arteriosus
    B. Ductus venosus
    C. Aorta
    D. Foramen ovale

26. Which of the following is *not* an artery?
    A. Femoral
    B. Popliteal
    C. Coronary
    D. Inferior vena cava

▶ *If you have had difficulty with this section, review pages 444-448.*

BLOOD PRESSURE
PULSE

If the statement is true, write "T" in the answer blank. If the statement is false, correct the statement by circling the incorrect term and inserting the correct term in the answer blank.

_____ 27. Blood pressure is highest in the veins and lowest in the arteries.

_____ 28. The difference between two blood pressures is referred to as *blood pressure deficit*.

_____ 29. If the blood pressure in the arteries were to decrease so that it became equal to the average pressure in the arterioles, circulation would increase.

_____ 30. A stroke is often the result of low blood pressure.

_____ 31. Massive hemorrhage increases blood pressure.

_____ 32. Blood pressure is the volume of blood in the vessels.

_____ 33. Both the strength and the rate of heartbeat affect cardiac output and blood pressure.

_____ 34. The diameter of the arterioles helps to determine how much blood drains out of arteries into arterioles.

_____ 35. A stronger heartbeat tends to decrease blood pressure and a weaker heartbeat tends to increase it.

_____ 36. The systolic pressure is the pressure while the ventricles relax.

_____ 37. The diastolic pressure is the pressure while the ventricles contract.

_____ 38. A device called a *sphygmomanometer* is used to measure blood pressures in clinical situations.

_____ 39. Loud, tapping Korotkoff sounds suddenly begin when the cuff pressure measured by the mercury column equals the systolic pressure.

_____ 40. The venous blood pressure within the left atrium is called the *central venous pressure.*

_____ 41. The pulse is a vein expanding and then recoiling.

_____ 42. The radial artery is located at the wrist.

_____ 43. The common carotid artery is located in the neck along the front edge of the sternocleidomastoid muscle.

_____ 44. The artery located at the bend of the elbow and used for locating the pulse is the dorsalis pedis.

▶ *If you have had difficulty with this section, review pages 448-452.*

CIRCULATORY SHOCK

Fill in the blanks.

45. Complications of septicemia may result in _____
_____.

46. _____ _____ results from any type of heart failure.

47. An acute type of allergic reaction called _____ results in _____.

48. _____ _____ results from widespread dilation of blood vessels caused by an imbalance in autonomic stimulation of smooth muscles in vessel walls.

49. *Hypovolemia* means "_____ _____
_____."

50. A type of septic shock that results from staphylococcal infections that begin in the vagina of menstruating women and spread to the blood is _____
_____ _____.

 If you have had difficulty with this section, review pages 452-455.

UNSCRAMBLE THE WORDS

51. **STMESYCI**

52. **NULVEE**

53. **RYTREA**

54. **USLEP**

Take the circled letters, unscramble them, and fill in the statement.

How Noah survived the flood.

55.

APPLYING WHAT YOU KNOW

56. Mrs. Champlin was enjoying a picnic lunch one day when a bee suddenly flew down and stung her. Within seconds, Mrs. Champlin began to experience difficulty breathing, tachycardia, a decrease in blood pressure, and cyanosis. What is Mrs. Champlin experiencing?

57. Mr. Attanas was scheduled to undergo extensive surgery. His surgeon, Dr. Berger, requested that two units of blood be available for Mr. Attanas should he require them. What complication of surgery was Dr. Berger hoping to avoid?

58. Rochelle is a hairstylist who works long hours. Lately she has noticed that her feet are sore and edematous. What might be the cause of these symptoms? What advice could offer Rochelle some relief from these symptoms?

59. Mr. Almaguer returned from surgery in stable condition. The nurse noted that each time she took Mr. Almaguer's pulse and blood pressure, the pulse became higher and the blood pressure lower than the last time. What might be the cause?

60. Word Find

Can you find the 15 terms from this chapter that are listed below? Words may be spelled top to bottom, bottom to top, right to left, left to right, or diagonally.

```
Y  H  Y  S  I  S  O  B  M  O  R  H  T  A  R
L  A  C  I  L  I  B  M  U  O  A  Y  N  I  Y
E  E  S  Y  S  T  E  M  I  C  C  G  D  E  U
M  V  E  N  U  L  E  D  D  C  I  X  M  D  I
E  Y  M  U  I  R  T  A  R  N  L  E  C  G  Y
N  O  I  T  A  Z  I  R  A  L  O  P  E  D  N
U  D  L  A  T  R  O  P  C  I  T  A  P  E  H
S  I  U  K  M  U  E  T  O  E  S  L  U  P  U
R  P  N  F  Y  C  B  E  D  R  A  L  Z  P  J
D  S  A  H  T  I  T  V  N  L  I  I  B  D  W
Q  U  R  O  I  V  A  Q  E  O  D  A  K  R  K
K  C  R  M  P  G  A  I  G  N  D  D  Z  Y  J
Y  I  Y  R  I  N  E  A  F  Z  L  Q  S  P  X
S  R  M  I  C  C  Q  O  A  W  U  N  H  O  K
P  T  A  V  H  H  Z  L  H  I  J  J  X  K  Z
```

Angina pectoris	ECG	Systemic
Apex	Endocardium	Thrombosis
Atrium	Hepatic portal	Tricuspid
Depolarization	Pulse	Umbilical
Diastolic	Semilunar	Venule

DID YOU KNOW?

Every pound of excess fat contains 200 miles of additional capillaries.

CIRCULATION OF THE BLOOD

Fill in the crossword puzzle.

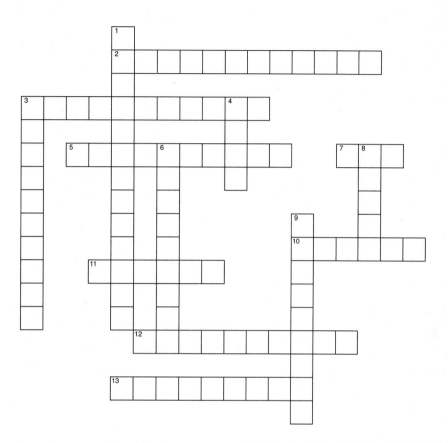

ACROSS

2. Inflammation of the lining of the heart
3. Bicuspid valve (two words)
5. Inner layer of pericardium
7. Cardiopulmonary resuscitation (abbreviation)
10. Carries blood away from the heart
11. Upper chamber of heart
12. Lower chambers of the heart
13. SA node

DOWN

1. Unique blood circulation through the liver (two words)
3. Muscular layer of the heart
4. Carries blood to the heart
6. Tiny artery
8. Heart rate
9. Carries blood from arterioles into venules

CHECK YOUR KNOWLEDGE

Multiple Choice

Circle the correct answer.

1. The medical term for high blood pressure is:
    A. Arteriosclerosis
    B. Cyanosis
    C. Hypertension
    D. Central venous pressure

2. Septic shock is caused by:
    A. Complications of toxins in the blood
    B. A nerve condition
    C. A drop in blood pressure
    D. Blood vessel dilation

3. Hypovolemic shock is caused by:
    A. Heart failure
    B. Dilated blood vessels
    C. A drop in blood volume
    D. A severe allergic reaction

4. Which vessels collect blood from the capillaries and return it to the heart?
    A. Arteries
    B. Sinuses
    C. Veins
    D. Arterioles

5. The innermost coat of an artery that comes into direct contact with blood is called the:
    A. Lumen
    B. Tunica externa
    C. Tunica intima
    D. Tunica media

6. Hemorrhoids can best be described as:
    A. Varicose veins
    B. Varicose veins in the rectum
    C. Thrombophlebitis of the rectum
    D. Clot formation in the rectum

7. In the fetal circulation:
    A. The ductus venosus allows most blood from the placenta to bypass the fetal liver.
    B. The umbilical vein carries oxygen-poor blood.
    C. The foramen ovale connects the aorta and the pulmonary artery.
    D. None of the above are true.

8. Which of the following events, if any, would *not* cause the blood pressure to increase?
    A. Hemorrhaging
    B. Increasing the viscosity of the blood
    C. Increasing the strength of the heartbeat
    D. All of the above

9. Arteriosclerosis is a disorder of the:
    A. Heart
    B. Veins
    C. Capillaries
    D. Arteries

10. A common type of vascular disease that occludes arteries by lipids and other matter is:
    A. Arteriosclerotic plaque
    B. Atherosclerosis
    C. Varicose veins
    D. Thrombophlebitis

Matching

Select the most appropriate answer from column B for each item in column A. (There is only one correct answer for each item.)

Column A

_____ 11. Largest artery
_____ 12. Decreased blood supply
_____ 13. Leg vein
_____ 14. Fetal circulation
_____ 15. Arterial procedure
_____ 16. Vein inflammation
_____ 17. Lung circulation
_____ 18. Weakened artery
_____ 19. Largest vein
_____ 20. Myocardial infarction

Column B

A. Ischemia
B. Phlebitis
C. Foramen ovale
D. Aneurysm
E. Vena cava
F. Angioplasty
G. Aorta
H. Pulmonary
I. Great saphenous vein
J. Cardiogenic shock

FETAL CIRCULATION

1. _____

2. _____

3. _____

4. _____

5. _____

6. _____

7. _____

8. _____

9. _____

10. _____

11. _____

12. _____

13. _____

14. _____

15. _____

16. _____

17. _____

18. _____

HEPATIC PORTAL CIRCULATION

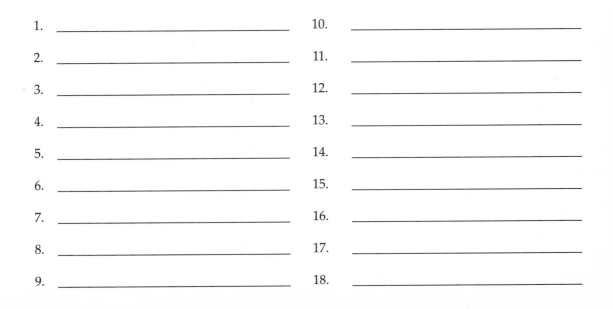

1. _____

2. _____

3. _____

4. _____

5. _____

6. _____

7. _____

8. _____

9. _____

10. _____

11. _____

12. _____

13. _____

14. _____

15. _____

16. _____

17. _____

18. _____

PRINCIPAL ARTERIES OF THE BODY

1. _____
2. _____
3. _____
4. _____
5. _____
6. _____
7. _____
8. _____
9. _____
10. _____
11. _____
12. _____
13. _____
14. _____
15. _____
16. _____
17. _____
18. _____
19. _____
20. _____
21. _____
22. _____
23. _____
24. _____
25. _____
26. _____
27. _____
28. _____
29. _____
30. _____

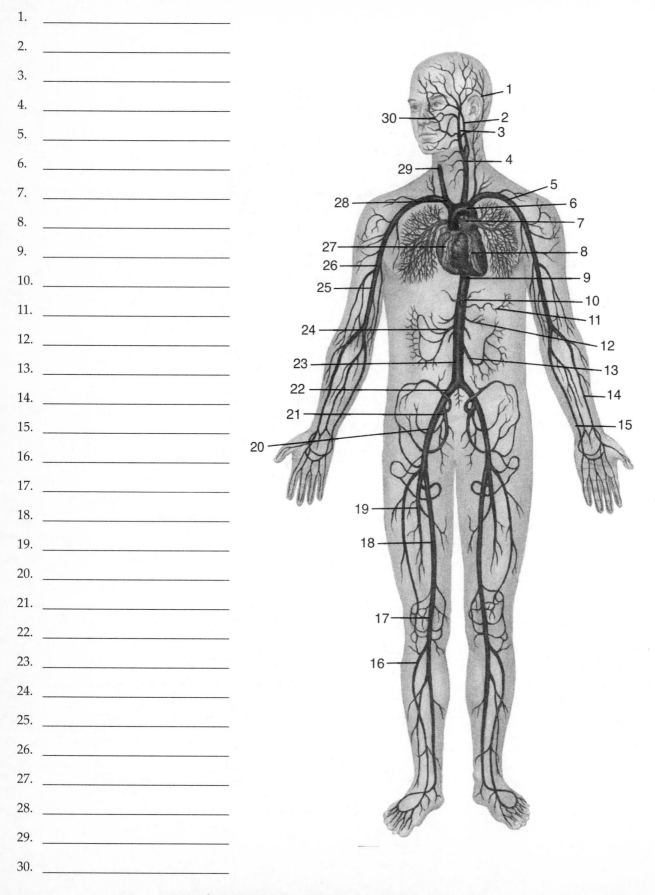

PRINCIPAL VEINS OF THE BODY

1. _____

2. _____

3. _____

4. _____

5. _____

6. _____

7. _____

8. _____

9. _____

10. _____

11. _____

12. _____

13. _____

14. _____

15. _____

16. _____

17. _____

18. _____

19. _____

20. _____

21. _____

22. _____

23. _____

24. _____

25. _____

26. _____

27. _____

28. _____

29. _____

30. _____

31. _____

32. _____

33. _____

34. _____

The Lymphatic System and Immunity

The lymphatic system is similar to the circulatory system. Lymph, like blood, flows through an elaborate route of vessels. In addition to lymphatic vessels, the lymphatic system consists of lymph nodes, lymph, and the spleen. Unlike the circulatory system, the lymphatic vessels do not form a closed circuit. Lymph flows only once through the vessels before draining into the general blood circulation. This system is a filtering mechanism for microorganisms and serves as a protective device against foreign invaders such as cancer.

The immune system is the armed forces division of the body. Ready to attack at a moment's notice, the immune system defends us against the major enemies of the body: microorganisms, foreign transplanted tissue cells, and our own cells that have turned malignant.

The most numerous cells of the immune system are the lymphocytes. These cells circulate in the body's fluids seeking invading organisms and destroying them with powerful lymphotoxins, lymphokines, or antibodies.

Phagocytes, another large group of immune system cells, assist with the destruction of foreign invaders by a process known as *phagocytosis*. Neutrophils, monocytes, and connective tissue cells called *macrophages* use this process to surround unwanted microorganisms and ingest and digest them, rendering them harmless to the body.

Another weapon that the immune system possesses is complement. Normally a group of inactive enzymes present in the blood, complement can be activated to kill invading cells by drilling holes in their cytoplasmic membranes, which allows fluid to enter the cell until it bursts.

Your review of this chapter will give you an understanding of how the body defends itself from the daily invasion of destructive substances.

TOPICS FOR REVIEW

Before progressing to Chapter 16 you should familiarize yourself with the functions of the lymphatic system, the immune system, and the major structures that make up these systems. Your review should include knowledge of lymphatic vessels, lymph nodes, lymph, antibodies, complement, and the development of B and T cells. Your study should also include the differences in humoral and cell-mediated immunity. Finally, an understanding of the excessive responses of the immune system and immune system deficiencies are necessary to complete your review of this chapter.

THE LYMPHATIC SYSTEM

Fill in the blanks.

1. _____ is a specialized fluid formed in the tissue spaces that will be transported by way of specialized vessels to eventually reenter the circulatory system.

2. Blood plasma that has filtered out of capillaries into microscopic spaces between cells is called _____ _____.

3. Tiny blind-ended tubes distributed in the tissue spaces are called _____ _____.

4. Lymph eventually empties into two terminal vessels called the _____ _____ _____ and the _____ _____.

5. The thoracic duct has an enlarged pouchlike structure called the _____ _____.

6. Lymph is filtered by moving through _____ _____, which are located in clusters along the pathway of lymphatic vessels.

7. Lymph enters the node through four _____ lymph vessels.

8. Lymph exits the node through a single _____ lymph vessel.

9. An abnormal condition in which tissues exhibit edema because of the accumulation of lymph is _____.

10. Hodgkin's disease is an example of _____.

▶ *If you have had difficulty with this section, review pages 462-467.*

THYMUS
TONSILS
SPLEEN

Choose the correct response.

A. Thymus   B. Tonsils   C. Spleen

_____ 11. Palatine, pharyngeal, and lingual are examples

_____ 12. The largest lymphoid organ in the body

_____ 13. Destroys worn-out red blood cells

_____ 14. Located in the mediastinum

_____ 15. Serves as a reservoir for blood

_____ 16. T-lymphocytes

_____ 17. Largest at puberty

▶ *If you have had difficulty with this section, review pages 467-468.*

THE IMMUNE SYSTEM

Match the term on the left with the proper selection on the right.

_____ 18.   Nonspecific immunity
_____ 19.   Inherited immunity
_____ 20.   Specific immunity
_____ 21.   Acquired immunity
_____ 22.   Immunization

A.   Inborn immunity
B.   Natural immunity
C.   General protection
D.   Artificial exposure
E.   Memory

IMMUNE SYSTEM MOLECULES

Match the term that applies to each of the following descriptions. Place the letter for the term in the appropriate answer blank.

_____ 23.   A type of very specific antibodies produced from a population of identical cells
_____ 24.   Protein compounds normally present in the body
_____ 25.   Also known as *antibody-mediated immunity*
_____ 26.   Combines with antibody to produce humoral immunity
_____ 27.   Antibody
_____ 28.   The process of changing antibody molecule shape slightly to expose binding sites
_____ 29.   Capable of producing large quantities of very specific antibodies
_____ 30.   Inactive proteins in blood

A.   Antibodies
B.   Antigen
C.   Monoclonal
D.   Complement fixation
E.   Complement
F.   Humoral
G.   Combining site
H.   Hybridomas

▶ *If you have had difficulty with this section, review pages 468-472.*

IMMUNE SYSTEM CELLS

Circle the correct answer.

31. The most numerous cells of the immune system are the:
   A.   Monocytes
   B.   Eosinophils
   C.   Neutrophils
   D.   Lymphocytes
   E.   Complement

32. The second stage of B cell development changes an immature B cell into a/an:
   A.   Plasma cell
   B.   Stem cell
   C.   Antibody
   D.   Activated B cell
   E.   Immature B cell

33. Which one of the following occurs last in the immune process?
   A.   Plasma cells
   B.   Stem cells
   C.   Antibodies
   D.   Activated B cells
   E.   Immature B cells

34. Which one of the following is part of the cell membrane of B cells?
   A.   Complement
   B.   Antigens
   C.   Antibodies
   D.   Epitopes
   E.   None of the above

35. Immature B cells have:
    A. Four types of defense mechanisms on their cell membrane
    B. Several kinds of defense mechanisms on their cell membrane
    C. One specific kind of defense mechanism on their cell membrane
    D. No defense mechanisms on their cell membrane

36. Development of an immature B cell depends on the B cell coming in contact with:
    A. Complement
    B. Antibodies
    C. Lymphotoxins
    D. Lymphokines
    E. Antigens

37. The kind of cell that produces large numbers of antibodies is the:
    A. B cell
    B. Stem cell
    C. T cell
    D. Memory cell
    E. Plasma cell

38. Just one of these short-lived cells that make antibodies can produce _____ of them per second.
    A. 20
    B. 200
    C. 2,000
    D. 20,000

39. Which of the following statements is *not* true of memory cells?
    A. They can secrete antibodies.
    B. They are found in lymph nodes.
    C. They develop into plasma cells.
    D. They can react with antigens.
    E. All of the above are true of memory cells.

40. T cell development begins in the:
    A. Lymph nodes
    B. Liver
    C. Pancreas
    D. Spleen
    E. Thymus

41. B cells function indirectly to produce:
    A. Humoral immunity
    B. Cell-mediated immunity
    C. Lymphotoxins
    D. Lymphokines

42. T cells function to produce:
    A. Humoral immunity
    B. Cell-mediated immunity
    C. Antibodies
    D. Memory cells

▶ *If you have had difficulty with this section, review pages 472-477.*

HYPERSENSITIVITY OF THE IMMUNE SYSTEM

Circle the correct answer.

43. The term *allergy* is used to describe (hypersensitivity or hyposensitivity) of the immune system to relatively harmless environmental antigens.

44. Antigens that trigger an allergic response are often called (antibodies or allergens).

45. (Anaphylactic shock or Urticaria) is a life-threatening condition.

46. A common autoimmune disease is (lupus or SCID).

47. Erythroblastosis fetalis is an example of (isoimmunity or autoimmunity).

48. The antigens most commonly involved in transplant rejection are called (SCIDs or HLAs).

▶ *If you have had difficulty with this section, review pages 477-479.*

IMMUNE DEFICIENCY

Select the correct response.

A. Congenital   B. Acquired (after birth)

_____ 49.   AIDS

_____ 50.   SCID

_____ 51.   Improper B cell development

_____ 52.   Viral infection

_____ 53.   Genetic defect

▶ *If you have had difficulty with this section, review pages 479-482.*

UNSCRAMBLE THE WORDS

54. **N T C M P E O L E M**

55. **M T M Y I U N I**

56. **O E N C L S**

57. **F N R O E R T E N I**

Take the circled letters, unscramble them, and fill in the statement.

...and please, don't let me forget to remember!

What the student was praying for the night before exams.

58.

APPLYING WHAT YOU KNOW

59. Two-year old baby Metcalfe was exposed to chickenpox and subsequently developed the disease. What type of immunity will be developed as a result of this?

60. Marcia was a bisexual and an intravenous drug user. She has developed a type of skin cancer known as Kaposi's sarcoma. What is Marcia's primary diagnosis?

61. Baby Wilson was born without a thymus gland. Immediate plans were made for a transplant to be performed. In the meantime, baby Wilson was placed in strict isolation. For what reason was he placed in isolation?

62. Word Find

Can you find the 14 terms from this chapter that are listed below? Words may be spelled top to bottom, bottom to top, right to left, left to right, or diagonally.

```
I  N  F  L  A  M  M  A  T  O  R  Y  F  C  G
Q  N  L  O  Y  Z  O  C  C  P  A  O  F  S  X
M  W  T  A  A  M  N  J  X  Q  K  R  N  P  H
U  R  L  E  R  M  P  X  B  R  U  I  A  L  C
C  M  A  C  R  O  P  H  A  G  E  I  E  D  Z
X  M  N  D  K  F  M  N  O  T  U  C  R  N  M
A  E  O  R  E  Z  E  U  O  C  F  B  Y  E  B
Y  P  L  E  B  G  G  R  H  T  Y  T  S  E  D
Y  S  C  R  I  S  P  J  O  E  I  T  M  L  A
Z  M  O  T  J  X  E  T  O  N  A  E  E  P  X
T  O  N  S  I  L  S  S  U  M  Y  H  T  S  Y
W  A  O  C  J  N  I  M  W  K  O  Z  E  N  D
D  W  M  K  W  R  M  O  I  P  S  H  Y  B  G
F  H  W  U  J  I  Z  F  V  D  Z  L  Y  T  X
```

Acquired	Interferon	Proteins
Antigen	Lymph	Spleen
Humoral	Lymphocytes	Thymus
Immunity	Macrophage	Tonsils
Inflammatory	Monoclonal	

DID YOU KNOW?

In the United States, the HIV infection rate is increasing four times faster in women than in men. Women tend to underestimate their risk.

Ten percent of all HIV/AIDS cases are individuals 50 years of age and older.

LYMPH AND IMMUNITY

Fill in the crossword puzzle.

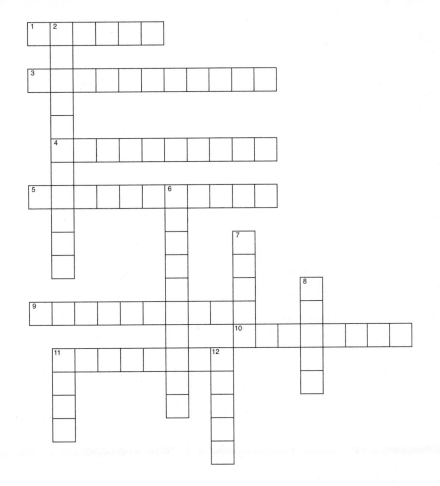

ACROSS

1. Largest lymphoid organ in the body
3. Connective tissue cells that are phagocytes
4. Protein compounds normally present in the body
5. Remain in reserve then turn into plasma cells when needed (two words)
9. Synthetically produced to fight certain diseases
10. Lymph exits the node through this lymph vessel
11. Lymph enters the node through these lymph vessels

DOWN

2. Secretes a copious amount of antibodies into the blood (two words)
6. Inactive proteins
7. Family of identical cells descended from one cell
8. Type of lymphocyte (humoral immunity—two words)
11. Immune deficiency disorder
12. Type of lymphocyte (cell-mediated immunity—two words)

CHECK YOUR KNOWLEDGE

Multiple Choice

Circle the correct answer.

1. T cells do which of the following?
   A. Develop in the thymus
   B. Form memory cells
   C. Form plasma cells
   D. All of the above

2. Lymph does which of the following?
   A. Forms as blood plasma filters out of capillaries
   B. Empties into the heart
   C. Flows through lymphatic arteries
   D. All of the above

3. Acquired immune deficiency syndrome is characterized by which of the following?
   A. Caused by a retrovirus
   B. Causes inadequate T cell formation
   C. Can result in death from cancer or infection
   D. All of the above

4. Interferon is:
   A. Produced by B cells
   B. A protein compound that protects other cells by interfering with the ability of a virus to reproduce
   C. A group of inactive enzyme proteins normally present in blood
   D. All of the above

5. B cells do which of the following?
   A. Develop into plasma cells and memory cells
   B. Establish humoral immunity
   C. Develop from primitive cells in bone marrow called *stem cells*
   D. All of the above

6. Which of the following functions to kill invading cells by drilling a hole in the plasma membrane?
   A. Interferon
   B. Complement
   C. Antibody
   D. Memory cell

7. Which of the following cell types function in the immune system?
   A. Macrophages
   B. Lymphocytes
   C. T cells
   D. All of the above

8. Which of the following is an example of phagocytes?
   A. Kupffer's cells
   B. Dust cells
   C. Macrophages
   D. All of the above

9. What is a rapidly growing population of identical cells that produce large quantities of specific antibodies called?
   A. Complementary
   B. Lymphotoxic
   C. Chemotactic
   D. Monoclonal

10. Which of the following is a form of passive natural immunity?
    A. A child develops measles and acquires an immunity to subsequent infection.
    B. Antibodies are injected into an infected individual.
    C. An infant receives protection through its mother's milk.
    D. Vaccinations are given against smallpox.

Matching

Select the most correct answer from column B for each statement in column A. (Only one answer is correct.)

Column A

_____ 11. Adenoids
_____ 12. B cell
_____ 13. Clone
_____ 14. HIV virus
_____ 15. Complement
_____ 16. Filtration
_____ 17. Cisterna chyli
_____ 18. T cell
_____ 19. Vaccination
_____ 20. Antigen

Column B

A. Thoracic duct
B. Lymph node
C. Artificial immunity
D. Humoral immunity
E. Pharyngeal tonsils
F. Foreign protein
G. Inactive proteins
H. AIDS
I. Identical cells
J. Cell-mediated immunity

PRINCIPAL ORGANS OF THE LYMPHATIC SYSTEM

1. _____

2. _____

3. _____

4. _____

5. _____

6. _____

7. _____

8. _____

9. _____

10. _____

11. _____

12. _____

The Respiratory System

As you sit reviewing this system, your body needs 16 quarts of air per minute. Walking requires 24 quarts of air, and running requires 50 quarts per minute. The respiratory system provides the air necessary for you to perform your daily activities and eliminates the waste gases from the air that you breathe. Take a deep breath, and think of the air as entering some 250 million tiny air sacs similar in appearance to clusters of grapes. These microscopic air sacs expand to let air in and contract to force it out. These tiny sacs, or alveoli, are the functioning units of the respiratory system. They provide the necessary volume of oxygen and eliminate carbon dioxide 24 hours a day.

Air enters either through the mouth or the nasal cavity. It next passes through the pharynx and past the epiglottis, through the glottis and the rest of the larynx. It then continues down the trachea, into the bronchi to the bronchioles, and finally through the alveoli. The reverse occurs for expelled air.

The exchange of gases between air in the lungs and in the blood is known as *external respiration*. The exchange of gases that occurs between the blood and the cells of the body is known as *internal respiration*. By constantly supplying adequate oxygen and removing carbon dioxide as it forms, the respiratory system helps to maintain an environment conducive to maximum cell efficiency.

Your review of this system is necessary to provide you with an understanding of this essential homeostatic mechanism.

TOPICS FOR REVIEW

Before progressing to Chapter 17, you should have an understanding of the structure and function of the organs of the respiratory system. Your review should include knowledge of the mechanisms responsible for both internal and external respiration. Your study should conclude with a knowledge of the volumes of air exchanged in pulmonary ventilation, an understanding of how respiration is regulated, and the common disorders of the respiratory tract.

STRUCTURAL PLAN
RESPIRATORY TRACTS
RESPIRATORY MUCOSA

Match the term with the definition.

_____ 1. Function of respiratory system

_____ 2. Pharynx

_____ 3. Passive transport process responsible for
            actual exchange of gases

_____ 4. Assists with the movement of mucus toward
            the pharynx

_____ 5. Barrier between the blood in the capillaries
            and the air in the alveolus

_____ 6. Lines the tubes of the respiratory tree

_____ 7. Terminal air sacs

_____ 8. Trachea

_____ 9. Surround alveoli

_____ 10. Homeostatic mechanism

A. Diffusion

B. Respiratory membrane

C. Alveoli

D. Capillaries

E. Respiration

F. Respiratory mucosa

G. Upper respiratory tract

H. Lower respiratory tract

I. Cilia

J. Air distributor

Fill in the blanks.

The organs of the respiratory system are designed to perform two basic functions. They serve as an

(11) _____ _____ and as a

(12) _____ _____. In addition to the

above, the respiratory system (13) _____,

(14) _____, and (15) _____ the air we

breathe. Respiratory organs include the (16) _____,

(17) _____, (18) _____,

(19) _____, (20) _____, and the

(21) _____. The respiratory system ends in millions of tiny, thin-walled sacs

called (22) _____. (23) _____ of gases

takes place in these sacs. Two aspects of the structure of these sacs assist them in the exchange of gases. First,

an extremely thin membrane, the (24) _____

_____, allows for easy exchange, and second, the large number of air sacs

makes an enormous (25) _____ area.

▷ *If you have had difficulty with this section, review pages 489-493.*

NOSE
PHARYNX
LARYNX
DISORDERS OF UPPER RESPIRATORY TRACT

Circle the word or phrase that does not belong.

26. Nares   Septum   Oropharynx   Conchae

27. Conchae   Frontal   Maxillary   Sphenoidal

28. Oropharynx   Throat   5 inches   Epiglottis

29. Pharyngeal   Adenoids   Uvula   Nasopharynx

30. Middle ear   Tubes   Nasopharynx   Larynx

31. Voice box   Thyroid cartilage Tonsils   Vocal cords

32. Palatine   Eustachian tube   Tonsils   Oropharynx

33. Pharynx   Epiglottis   Adam's apple   Voice box

Choose the correct response.

A. Nose   B. Pharynx   C. Larynx

_____ 34. Warms and humidifies air

_____ 35. Air and food pass through here

_____ 36. Sinuses

_____ 37. Conchae

_____ 38. Septum

_____ 39. Tonsils

_____ 40. Middle ear infections

_____ 41. Epiglottis

_____ 42. Rhinitis

_____ 43. Sore throat

_____ 44. Epistaxis

▶ *If you have had difficulty with this section, review pages 493-500.*

TRACHEA
BRONCHI, BRONCHIOLES, AND ALVEOLI
LUNGS AND PLEURA

Fill in the blanks.

45. The windpipe is more properly referred to as the _____.

46. _____ keep the framework of the trachea almost noncollapsible.

47. A life-saving technique designed to free the trachea of ingested food or foreign objects is the
_____ _____.

48. The first branch or division of the trachea leading to the lungs is the _____
_____.

49. Each alveolar duct ends in several _____
_____.

50. The narrow part of each lung, up under the collarbone, is its _____.

51. The _____ covers the outer surface of the lungs and lines the inner surface of the rib cage.

52. Inflammation of the lining of the thoracic cavity is _____.

53. The presence of air in the pleural space on one side of the chest is a _____.

▷ *If you have had difficulty with this section, review pages 500-506.*

RESPIRATION

If the statement is true, write "T" in the answer blank. If the statement is false, correct the statement by circling the incorrect term and inserting the correct term in the answer blank.

_____ 54. Diffusion is the process that moves air into and out of the lungs.

_____ 55. For inspiration to take place, the diaphragm and other respiratory muscles relax.

_____ 56. Diffusion is a passive process that results in movement up a concentration gradient.

_____ 57. The exchange of gases that occurs between blood in tissue capillaries and the body cells is external respiration.

_____ 58. Many pulmonary volumes can be measured as a person breathes into a spirometer.

_____ 59. Ordinarily we take about 2 pints of air into our lungs.

_____ 60. The amount of air normally breathed in and out with each breath is called *tidal volume.*

_____ 61. The largest amount of air that one can breathe out in one expiration is called *residual volume.*

_____ 62. The inspiratory reserve volume is the amount of air that can be forcibly inhaled after a normal inspiration.

▷ *If you have had difficulty with this section, review pages 506-510.*

Circle the correct answer.

63. The term that means the same thing as breathing is:
    A. Gas exchange
    B. Respiration
    C. Inspiration
    D. Expiration
    E. Pulmonary ventilation

64. Carbaminohemoglobin is formed when _____ bind(s) to hemoglobin.
    A. Oxygen
    B. Amino acids
    C. Carbon dioxide
    D. Nitrogen
    E. None of the above

65. Most of the oxygen transported by the blood is:
    A. Dissolved to white blood cells
    B. Bound to white blood cells
    C. Bound to hemoglobin
    D. Bound to carbaminohemoglobin
    E. None of the above

66. Which of the following does *not* occur during inspiration?
    A. Elevation of the ribs
    B. Elevation of the diaphragm
    C. Contraction of the diaphragm
    D. Chest cavity becomes longer from top to bottom

67. A young adult male would have a vital capacity of about _____ ml.
    A. 500
    B. 1,200
    C. 3,300
    D. 4,800
    E. 6,200

68. The amount of air that can be forcibly exhaled after expiring the tidal volume is known as the:
    A. Total lung capacity
    B. Vital capacity
    C. Inspiratory reserve volume
    D. Expiratory reserve volume
    E. None of the above

69. Which one of the following is correct?
    A. VC = TV - IRV + ERV
    B. VC = TV + IRV - ERV
    C. VC = TV + IRV × ERV
    D. VC = TV + IRV + ERV
    E. None of the above

▷ *If you have had difficulty with this section, review pages 506-510.*

REGULATION OF RESPIRATION
RECEPTORS INFLUENCING RESPIRATION
TYPES OF BREATHING

Match the term on the left with the proper selection on the right.

_____ 70. Inspiratory center
_____ 71. Chemoreceptors
_____ 72. Pulmonary stretch receptors
_____ 73. Dyspnea
_____ 74. Respiratory arrest
_____ 75. Eupnea

_____ 76. Hypoventilation

A. Difficult breathing
B. Located in carotid bodies
C. Slow and shallow respirations
D. Normal respiratory rate
E. Located in the medulla
F. Failure to resume breathing following a period of apnea
G. Located throughout pulmonary airways and in the alveoli

▷ *If you have had difficulty with this section, review pages 510-514.*

DISORDERS OF THE LOWER RESPIRATORY TRACT

Fill in the blanks.

77. _____ is an acute inflammation of the lungs in which the alveoli and bronchi become plugged with thick fluid.

78. _____ is still a major cause of death in many poor, densely populated regions of the world. It has recently reemerged as an important health problem in some major U.S. cities.

79. _____ may result from the progression of chronic bronchitis or other conditions as air becomes trapped within alveoli, causing them to enlarge and eventually rupture.

80. _____ is an obstructive disorder characterized by recurring spasms of the smooth muscle in the walls of the bronchial air passages.

▶ *If you have had difficulty with this section, review pages 514-517.*

UNSCRAMBLE THE WORDS

81. **SPUELIRY**

82. **CRNBOSITHI**

83. **SESXPTIAI**

84. **DDNEAOIS**

Take the circled letters, unscramble them, and fill in the statement.

What Mona Lisa was to DaVinci.

85.

APPLYING WHAT YOU KNOW

86. Mr. Gorski is a heavy smoker. Recently he has noticed that when he gets up in the morning, he has a bothersome cough that brings up a large accumulation of mucus. This cough persists for several minutes and then leaves until the next morning. What is an explanation for this problem?

87. Kim is 5 years old and is a mouth breather. She has repeated episodes of tonsillitis and the pediatrician, Dr. Smith, suggests removal of her tonsils and adenoids. He further suggests that the surgery will probably cure her mouth breathing problem. Why is this a possibility?

88. Ms. Peace developed emphysema. This disease reduces the capacity of the lungs to recoil elastically. Which respiratory air volumes will this condition affect? Why?

89. Word Find

Can you find the 14 terms from this chapter that are listed below? Words may be spelled top to bottom, bottom to top, right to left, left to right, or diagonally.

```
N  K  S  A  Q  B  I  L  V  A  D  T  I  X  D
O  X  O  O  B  F  I  F  G  I  M  N  R  G  Y
I  G  N  X  W  D  E  E  F  L  B  A  U  T  S
T  B  K  Y  N  H  E  F  O  I  U  T  I  R  P
A  T  M  H  E  O  U  T  R  C  C  C  P  V  N
L  L  A  E  P  S  I  R  I  Z  A  A  N  F  E
I  P  T  M  I  H  G  T  I  P  R  F  P  C  A
T  U  B  O  G  Q  E  V  A  Q  O  R  V  N  W
N  L  N  G  L  R  J  C  C  R  T  U  P  D  C
E  M  U  L  O  V  L  A  U  D  I  S  E  R  E
V  O  V  O  T  A  N  G  J  E  D  P  Z  U  U
O  N  K  B  T  C  N  U  U  E  B  O  S  J  S
P  A  L  I  I  K  E  U  C  N  O  Z  K  N  A
Y  R  V  N  S  D  I  O  N  E  D  A  M  F  I
H  Y  O  M  L  O  A  Z  D  T  Y  M  N  L  K
```

Adenoids	Epiglottis	Residual volume
Carotid body	Hypoventilation	Surfactant
Cilia	Inspiration	URI
Diffusion	Oxyhemoglobin	Vital capacity
Dyspnea	Pulmonary	

DID YOU KNOW?

If the alveoli in our lungs were flattened out they would cover one-half of a tennis court.

Eighty percent of lung cancer cases are due to cigarette smoking.

RESPIRATORY SYSTEM

Fill in the crossword puzzle.

ACROSS

1. Device used to measure the amount of air exchanged in breathing
6. Expiratory reserve volume (abbreviation)
7. Sphenoidal (two words)
8. Terminal air sacs
9. Shelflike structures that protrude into the nasal cavity
11. Inflammation of pleura
12. Respirations stop

DOWN

2. Surgical procedure to remove tonsils
3. Doctor who developed life-saving technique
4. Windpipe
5. Trachea branches into right and left structures
10. Voice box

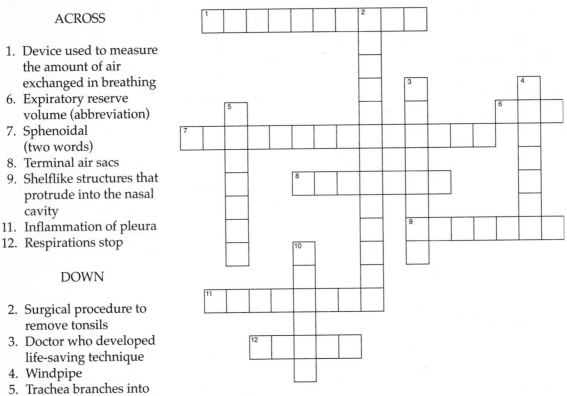

CHECK YOUR KNOWLEDGE

Multiple Choice

Circle the correct answer.

1. Chemoreceptors in the carotid and aortic bodies are characterized by which of the following?
   A. Sensitive to increases in blood carbon dioxide level
   B. Found in the brain
   C. Sensitive to increases in blood oxygen level
   D. Send impulses to the heart

2. What is the lowest segment of the pharynx called?
   A. Oropharynx
   B. Laryngopharynx
   C. Nasopharynx
   D. Hypopharynx

3. What is the narrow upper portion of a lung called?
   A. Base
   B. Notch
   C. Costal surface
   D. Apex

4. What is the largest amount of air that we can breathe in and out in one inspiration and expiration called?
   A. Tidal volume
   B. Vital capacity
   C. Residual volume
   D. Inspiratory reserve volume

5. Which of the following statements, if any, is *not* characteristic of human lungs?
   A. Both right and left lungs are composed of three lobes.
   B. Bronchi subdivide to form bronchioles.
   C. Capillary supply is abundant to facilitate gas exchange.
   D. All of the above statements are characteristic of human lungs.

6. Which body function is made possible by the existence of fibrous bands stretched across the larynx?
   A. Swallowing
   B. Breathing
   C. Diffusion
   D. Speech

7. The trachea is made almost noncollapsible by the presence of which of the following?
   A. Rings of cartilage
   B. Thyroid cartilage
   C. Epiglottis
   D. Vocal cords

8. Which of the following is true of the exchange of respiratory gases between lungs and blood?
   A. It takes place by diffusion.
   B. It is called *external respiration.*
   C. Both A and B are true.
   D. None of the above is true.

9. When the diaphragm contracts, which phase of ventilation is taking place?
   A. External respiration
   B. Expiration
   C. Internal respiration
   D. Inspiration

10. Which of the following is *not* characteristic of the nasal cavities?
    A. They contain many blood vessels that warm incoming air.
    B. They contain the adenoids.
    C. They are lined with mucous membranes.
    D. They are separated by a partition called the *nasal septum.*

Matching

Select the most correct answer from column B for each item in column A. (Only one answer is correct.)

Column A
_____ 11. Vocal cords
_____ 12. Pulmonary ventilation
_____ 13. Pleura
_____ 14. Pneumothorax
_____ 15. Emphysema
_____ 16. Throat
_____ 17. Ethmoidal
_____ 18. Windpipe
_____ 19. Alveoli
_____ 20. Surfactant

Column B
A. Serous membrane
B. Pharynx
C. Paranasal sinus
D. LVRS
E. Larynx
F. Diffusion
G. Collapsed lung
H. Trachea
I. Breathing
J. IRDS

SAGITTAL VIEW OF FACE AND NECK

1. _____
2. _____
3. _____
4. _____
5. _____
6. _____
7. _____
8. _____
9. _____
10. _____
11. _____

12. _____
13. _____
14. _____
15. _____
16. _____
17. _____
18. _____
19. _____
20. _____
21. _____
22. _____

RESPIRATORY ORGANS

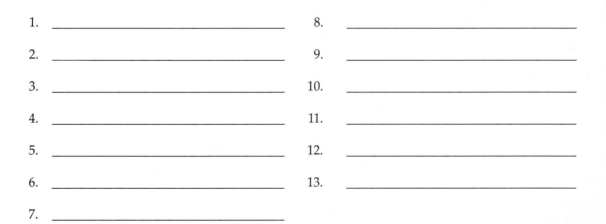

1. _____   8. _____

2. _____   9. _____

3. _____   10. _____

4. _____   11. _____

5. _____   12. _____

6. _____   13. _____

7. _____

PULMONARY VENTILATION VOLUMES

1 _____   6 _____ Vital capacity

1. _____   4. _____

2. _____   5. _____

3. _____

CHAPTER 17

The Digestive System

T hink of the last meal you ate. Imagine the different shapes, sizes, tastes, and textures that you so recently enjoyed. Think of those items circulating in your bloodstream in those same original shapes and sizes. Impossible? Of course! Because of this impossibility, you can begin to understand and marvel at the close relationship of the digestive system to the circulatory system. It is the digestive system that changes our food, both mechanically and chemically, into a form that is acceptable to the blood and the body.

This change begins the moment you take the very first bite. Digestion starts in the mouth, where food is chewed and mixed with saliva. It then moves down the pharynx and esophagus by peristalsis and enters the stomach. In the stomach it is churned and mixed with gastric juices to become chyme. The chyme goes from the stomach into the duodenum where it is further broken down chemically by intestinal fluids, bile, and pancreatic juice. Those secretions prepare the food for absorption all along the course of the small intestine. Products that are not absorbed pass on through the entire length of the small intestine (duodenum, jejunum, ileum). From there they enter into the cecum of the large intestine, the ascending colon, transverse colon, descending colon, sigmoid colon, into the rectum, and out the anus.

Products that are used in the cells undergo absorption. Absorption allows newly processed nutrients to pass through the walls of the digestive tract and into the bloodstream to be distributed to the cells.

Your review of this system will help you understand the mechanical and chemical processes necessary to convert food into energy sources and compounds necessary for survival.

TOPICS FOR REVIEW

Before progressing to Chapter 18, you should review the structure and function of all the organs of digestion. You should have an understanding of the process of digestion, both chemical and mechanical, and of the processes of absorption and metabolism.

THE DIGESTIVE SYSTEM
ORGANS OF THE DIGESTIVE SYSTEM

Fill in the blanks.

1. The organs of the digestive system form an irregular-shaped tube called the *alimentary canal* or
   _____ _____.

2. The churning of food in the stomach is an example of the _____ breakdown of food.

3. _____ breakdown occurs when digestive enzymes act on food as it passes through the digestive tract.

4. Waste material resulting from the digestive process is known as _____.

5. Foods undergo three kinds of processing in the body: _____, _____, and _____.

Select the correct response from the two choices given and insert the letter in the answer blank.

A. Main organ   B. Accessory organ

_____ 6.   Mouth

_____ 7.   Parotids

_____ 8.   Liver

_____ 9.   Stomach

_____ 10. Cecum

_____ 11. Esophagus

_____ 12. Rectum

_____ 13. Pharynx

_____ 14. Appendix

_____ 15. Teeth

_____ 16. Gallbladder

_____ 17. Pancreas

▶ *If you have had difficulty with this section, review pages 527-529.*

MOUTH

TEETH

SALIVARY GLANDS

Circle the correct answer.

18. Which one of the following is *not* a part of the roof of the mouth?
    A. Uvula
    B. Palatine bones
    C. Maxillary bones
    D. Soft palate
    E. All of the above are part of the roof of the mouth

19. The largest of the papillae on the surface of the tongue are the:
    A. Filiform
    B. Fungiform
    C. Vallate
    D. Taste buds

20. The first baby tooth, on an average, appears at:
    A. 2 months
    B. 1 year
    C. 3 months
    D. 1 month
    E. 6 months

21. The portion of the tooth that is covered with enamel is the:
    A. Pulp cavity
    B. Neck
    C. Root
    D. Crown
    E. None of the above is correct

22. The wall of the pulp cavity is surrounded by:
    A. Enamel
    B. Dentin
    C. Cementum
    D. Connective tissue
    E. Blood and lymphatic vessels

23. Which of the following teeth is missing from the deciduous arch?
    A. Central incisor
    B. Canine
    C. Second premolar
    D. First molar
    E. Second molar

24. The permanent central incisor erupts between the ages of _____.
    A. 9 and 13
    B. 5 and 6
    C. 7 and 10
    D. 7 and 8
    E. None of the above

25. The third molar appears between the ages of
    _____.
    A. 10 and 14
    B. 5 and 8
    C. 11 and 16
    D. 17 and 24
    E. None of the above

26. A general term for infection of the gums is:
    A. Dental caries
    B. Leukoplakia
    C. Vincent's angina
    D. Gingivitis

27. The ducts of the _____ glands open into the floor of the mouth.
    A. Sublingual
    B. Submandibular
    C. Parotid
    D. Carotid

28. The volume of saliva secreted per day is about:
    A. One-half pint
    B. One pint
    C. One liter
    D. One gallon

29. Mumps are an infection of the:
    A. Parotid gland
    B. Sublingual gland
    C. Submandibular gland
    D. Tonsils

30. Incisors are used during mastication to:
    A. Cut
    B. Piece
    C. Tear
    D. Grind

31. Another name for the third molar is:
    A. Central incisor
    B. Wisdom tooth
    C. Canine
    D. Lateral incisor

32. After food has been chewed, it is formed into a small rounded mass called a:
    A. Moat
    B. Chyme
    C. Bolus
    D. Protease

▶ *If you have had difficulty with this section, review pages 529-536.*

WALL OF DIGESTIVE TRACT

Fill in the blanks.

33. The serosa of the digestive tube is composed of the _____ _____ in the abdominal cavity.

34. The digestive tract extends from the _____ to the _____.

35. The inside or hollow space within the alimentary canal is called the _____.

36. The inside layer of the digestive tract is the _____.

37. The connective tissue layer that lies beneath the lining of the digestive tract is the _____.

38. The muscularis contracts and moves food through the gastrointestinal tract by a process known as
_____.

39. The outermost covering of the digestive tube is the _____.

40. The loops of the digestive tract are anchored to the posterior wall of the abdominal cavity by the
_____.

PHARYNX
ESOPHAGUS
STOMACH

Fill in the blanks.

The (41) _____ is a tubelike structure that functions as part of both respiratory and digestive systems. It connects the mouth with the (42) _____. The esophagus serves as a passageway for movement of food from the pharynx to the
(43) _____. Food enters the stomach by passing through the muscular
(44) _____ _____ at the end of the esophagus. Contraction of the stomach mixes the food thoroughly with the gastric juices and breaks it down into a semisolid mixture called (45) _____. The three divisions of the stomach are the (46) _____, (47) _____, and
(48) _____. Food is held in the stomach by the
(49) _____ _____ muscle long enough for partial digestion to occur. After food has been in the stomach for approximately 3 hours, the chyme will enter the (50) _____ _____.

Match the term with the correct definition.

_____ 51.   Stomach folds

_____ 52.   Upper right border of stomach

_____ 53.   Heartburn

_____ 54.   10-inch passageway

_____ 55.   Shown to be an effective treatment of Crohn's disease

_____ 56.   Semisolid mixture of stomach contents

_____ 57.   Muscle contractions of the digestive system

_____ 58.   Craterlike wound in digestive system caused by tissue destruction

_____ 59.   Stomach pushes through the gap in the diaphragm

_____ 60.   Lower left border of stomach

A.   Esophagus
B.   Chyme
C.   Peristalsis
D.   Rugae
E.   Ulcer
F.   Greater curvature
G.   Acid indigestion
H.   Triple therapy
I.   Hiatal hernia
J.   Lesser curvature

▶ *If you have had difficulty with this section, review pages 536-542.*

SMALL INTESTINE
LIVER AND GALLBLADDER
PANCREAS

Circle the correct answer.

61. Which one is *not* part of the small intestine?
    A. Jejunum
    B. Ileum
    C. Cecum
    D. Duodenum

62. Which one of the following structures does *not* increase the surface area of the intestine for absorption?
    A. Plicae
    B. Rugae
    C. Villi
    D. Brush border

63. The union of the cystic duct and hepatic duct form the:
    A. Common bile duct
    B. Major duodenal papilla
    C. Minor duodenal papilla
    D. Pancreatic duct

64. Obstruction of the _____ will lead to jaundice.
    A. Hepatic duct
    B. Pancreatic duct
    C. Cystic duct
    D. None of the above

65. Each villus in the intestine contains a lymphatic vessel or _____ that serves to absorb lipid or fat materials from the chyme.
    A. Plica
    B. Lacteal
    C. Villa
    D. Microvilli

66. The middle third of the duodenum contains the:
    A. Islets
    B. Fundus
    C. Body
    D. Rugae
    E. Major duodenal papilla

67. Cholelithiasis is the term used to describe:
    A. Biliary colic
    B. Jaundice
    C. Portal hypertension
    D. Gall stones

68. The liver is an:
    A. Enzyme
    B. Endocrine organ
    C. Endocrine gland
    D. Exocrine gland

69. Fats in chyme stimulate the secretion of the hormone:
    A. Lipase
    B. Cholecystokinin
    C. Protease
    D. Amylase

70. The largest gland in the body is the:
    A. Pituitary
    B. Thyroid
    C. Liver
    D. Thymus

 If you have had difficulty with this section, review pages 542-547.

LARGE INTESTINE
APPENDIX
PERITONEUM

If the statement is true, write "T" in the answer blank. If the statement is false, correct the statement by circling the incorrect term and inserting the correct term in the answer blank.

_____ 71. Bacteria in the large intestine are responsible for the synthesis of vitamin E needed for normal blood clotting.

_____ 72. Villi in the large intestine absorb salts and water.

_____ 73. If waste products pass rapidly through the large intestine, constipation results.

_____ 74. The ileocecal valve opens into the sigmoid colon.

_____ 75. The splenic flexure is the bend between the ascending colon and the transverse colon.

_____ 76. The splenic colon is the S-shaped segment that terminates in the rectum.

_____ 77. The appendix serves no important digestive function in humans.

_____ 78. For patients with suspected appendicitis, a physician will often evaluate the appendix by a digital rectal examination.

_____ 79. The visceral layer of the peritoneum lines the abdominal cavity.

_____ 80. The greater omentum is shaped like a fan and serves to anchor the small intestine to the posterior abdominal wall.

_____ 81. Diarrhea is an inflammation of abnormal saclike outpouchings of the intestinal wall.

_____ 82. Crohn's disease is a type of autoimmune colitis.

_____ 83. A colostomy is a surgical procedure in which an artificial anus is created on the abdominal wall.

_____ 84. Peritonitis is the abnormal accumulation of fluid in the peritoneal space.

▶ *If you have had difficulty with this section, review pages 547-554.*

DIGESTION
ABSORPTION
METABOLISM

Circle the correct answer.

85. Which one of the following substances does *not* contain any enzymes?
    A. Saliva
    B. Bile
    C. Gastric juice
    D. Pancreatic juice
    E. Intestinal juice

86. Which one of the following is a simple sugar?
    A. Maltose
    B. Sucrose
    C. Lactose
    D. Glucose
    E. Starch

87. Cane sugar is the same as:
    A. Maltose
    B. Lactose
    C. Sucrose
    D. Glucose
    E. None of the above

88. Most of the digestion of carbohydrates takes
    place in the:
    A. Mouth
    B. Stomach
    C. Small intestine
    D. Large intestine

89. Fats are broken down into:
    A. Amino acids
    B. Simple sugars
    C. Fatty acids
    D. Disaccharides

▶ *If you have had difficulty with this section, review pages 554-556.*

CHEMICAL DIGESTION

90. Fill in the blank areas on the chart below.

DIGESTIVE JUICES AND ENZYMES	SUBSTANCE DIGESTED (OR HYDROLYZED)	RESULTING PRODUCT
Saliva		
1. Amylase	1.	1. Maltose
Gastric Juice		
2. Protease (pepsin) plus hydrochloric acid	2. Proteins	2.
Pancreatic Juice		
3. Protease (trypsin)	3. Proteins (intact or partially digested)	3.
4. Lipase	4.	4. Fatty acids, monoglycerides, and glycerol
5. Amylase	5.	5. Maltose
Intestinal Juice		
6. Peptidases	6.	6. Amino acids
7.	7. Sucrose	7. Glucose and fructose
8. Lactase	8.	8. Glucose and galactose (simple sugars)
9. Maltase	9. Maltose	9.

▶ *If you have had difficulty with this section, review page 555.*

UNSCRAMBLE THE WORDS

91. **S L B O U**

☐ ◯ ◯ ☐

92. **E Y C H M**

◯ ☐ ☐ ◯

93. **L L A A P P I**

☐ ◯ ☐ ☐ ☐ ◯

94. **P M E R T E U I O N**

◯ ☐ ◯ ☐ ☐ ◯ ☐ ☐ ☐

Take the circled letters, unscramble them, and fill in the statement.

What the groom gave his bride after the wedding.

95. ☐ ☐ ☐ ☐   ☐ ☐ ☐ ☐ ☐

APPLYING WHAT YOU KNOW

96. Mr. Amoto was a successful businessman, but he worked too hard and was always under great stress. He took high doses of aspirin, almost daily, to relieve his stress headaches. His doctor cautioned him that if he did not alter his style of living he would be subject to hyperacidity. What could be a result of hyperacidity?

97. Baby Nicholas has been regurgitating his bottle feeding at every meal. The milk is curdled, but does not appear to be digested. He has become dehydrated, and so his mother, Bobbi, is taking him to the pediatrician. What is a possible diagnosis from your textbook reading?

98. Mr. Lynch has high cholesterol and quickly lost 25 pounds on an ultra low-fat diet. He has recently noticed a yellowish cast to his skin and periodic pain in the right upper quadrant of the abdominopelvic region. What is a possible diagnosis for Mr. Lynch? What is the name of the surgical procedure that may be performed on Mr. Lynch?

99.   Word Find

Can you find the 22 terms from this chapter that are listed below? Words may be spelled top to bottom, bottom to top, right to left, left to right, or diagonally.

```
X M E T A B O L I S M X X W
R S D P E R I S T A L S I S
E V A M N O I T S E G I D R
E D E E U O Q T W Q O H N Q
Q Z H S R N I N T F E C E S
D H R E C C I T K C J A P E
Q W R N A T N V P Y R M P C
O C A T R B A P R H O A I
U Y I E O W T A P A O T W D
B O D R L N P B F Q J S V N
N T S Y F I S L U M E E B U
W G J A L U V U N R N W O A
Q S N L X D U O D E N U M J
H C A V I T Y M U C O S A D
Y E A A P H V W S V C Q J C
```

Absorption	Emulsify	Mucosa
Appendix	Feces	Pancreas
Cavity	Fundus	Papillae
Crown	Heartburn	Peristalsis
Dentin	Jaundice	Stomach
Diarrhea	Mastication	Uvula
Digestion	Mesentery	
Duodenum	Metabolism	

DID YOU KNOW?

The liver performs over 500 functions and produces over 1,000 enzymes to handle the chemical conversions necessary for survival.

About 20% of older adults have diabetes, and almost 40% have some impaired glucose tolerance.

DIGESTIVE SYSTEM

Fill in the crossword puzzle.

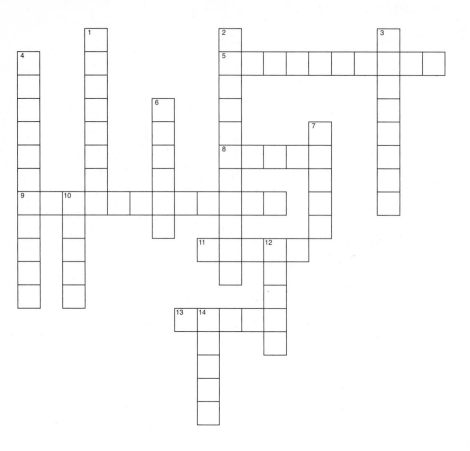

ACROSS

5. Digested food moves from intestine to blood
8. Semisolid mixture
9. Inflammation of the appendix
11. Rounded mass of food
13. Stomach folds

DOWN

1. Yellowish skin discoloration
2. Process of chewing
3. Fluid stools
4. Movement of food through digestive tract
6. Vomitus
7. Waste product of digestion
10. Intestinal folds
12. Open wound in digestive area acted on by acid juices
14. Prevents food from entering nasal cavities

CHECK YOUR KNOWLEDGE

Multiple Choice

Circle the correct answer.

1. During the process of digestion, *stored* bile is poured into the duodenum by which of the following?
   A. Gallbladder
   B. Liver
   C. Pancreas
   D. Spleen

2. The portion of the alimentary canal that mixes food with gastric juice and breaks it down into a mixture called *chyme*.
   A. Gallbladder
   B. Small intestine
   C. Stomach
   D. Large intestine

3. What is the middle portion of the small intestine called?
   A. Jejunum
   B. Ileum
   C. Duodenum
   D. Cecum

4. The crown of the tooth is covered externally with which of the following?
   A. Cementum
   B. Enamel
   C. Dentin
   D. Pulp

5. What is the layer of tissue that forms the outermost covering of organs found in the digestive tract called?
   A. Mucosa
   B. Serosa
   C. Submucosa
   D. Muscularis

6. Duodenal ulcers appear in which of the following?
   A. Stomach
   B. Small intestine
   C. Large intestine
   D. Esophagus

7. What is an extension of the peritoneum that is shaped like a giant pleated fan?
   A. Omentum
   B. Mesentery
   C. Peritoneal cavity
   D. Ligament

8. Protein digestion begins in the:
   A. Esophagus
   B. Small intestine
   C. Stomach
   D. Large intestine

9. The enzyme pepsin is concerned primarily with the digestion of which of the following?
   A. Sugars
   B. Starches
   C. Proteins
   D. Fats

10. The enzyme amylase converts which of the following?
    A. Starches to sugars
    B. Sugars to starches
    C. Proteins to amino acids
    D. Fatty acids and glycerol to fats

Completion

Complete the following statements using the terms listed below.

A. Ileum	G. Lower esophageal sphincter	M. Upper esophageal sphincter	S. Premolars
B. Amylase	H. Digestion	N. Sigmoid colon	T. Mucosa
C. Muscularis	I. Incisors	O. Canines	U. Submucosa
D. Metabolism	J. Greater omentum	P. Amino acids	V. Cecum
E. Cholecystokinin	K. Absorption	Q. Duodenum	W. Bile
F. Molars	L. Adventitia	R. Jejunum	X. Serosa

11. The S-shaped portion of the colon is called the _____.

12. The portion of the peritoneum that descends from the stomach and the transverse colon to form a lacy apron of fat over the intestines is called the _____.

13. The "building blocks" of protein molecules are _____.

14. The small intestine is made up of three sections called the _____, _____, and the _____.

15. Fats that enter into the digestive tract are emulsified when they are acted on by a substance called _____.

16. Foods undergo three kinds of processing in the body: _____, _____, and _____.

17. Fats in the chyme stimulate the secretion of _____, which stimulates contraction of the gallbladder to release bile.

18. The four tissue layers that make up the wall of the digestive tract are the _____, _____, _____, and _____.

19. Food enters the stomach by passing through a muscular structure at the end of the esophagus. This structure is called the _____.

20. The four major types of teeth found in the human mouth are _____, _____, _____, and _____.

LOCATION OF DIGESTIVE ORGANS

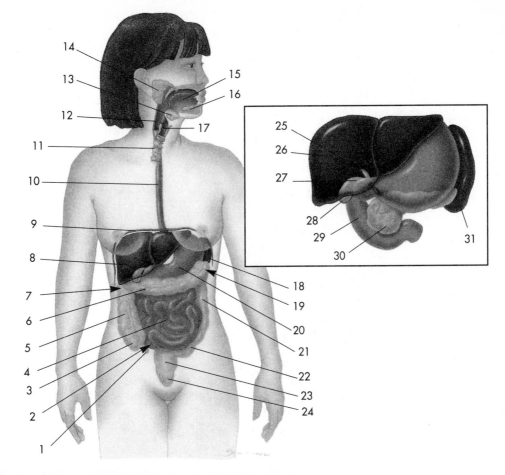

1. _____
2. _____
3. _____
4. _____
5. _____
6. _____
7. _____
8. _____
9. _____
10. _____
11. _____
12. _____
13. _____
14. _____
15. _____
16. _____

17. _____
18. _____
19. _____
20. _____
21. _____
22. _____
23. _____
24. _____
25. _____
26. _____
27. _____
28. _____
29. _____
30. _____
31. _____

TOOTH

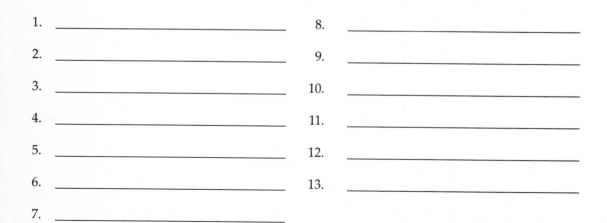

1. _____
2. _____
3. _____
4. _____
5. _____
6. _____
7. _____

8. _____
9. _____
10. _____
11. _____
12. _____
13. _____

THE SALIVARY GLANDS

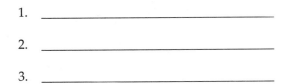

1. _____   4. _____

2. _____   5. _____

3. _____

STOMACH

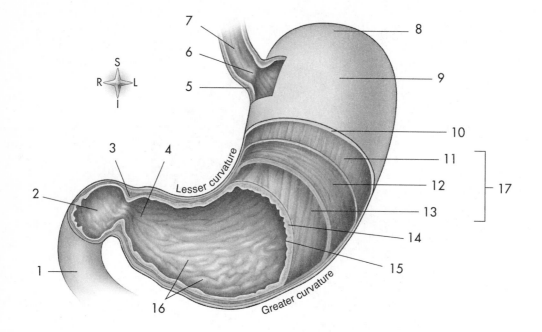

1. _____   10. _____

2. _____   11. _____

3. _____   12. _____

4. _____   13. _____

5. _____   14. _____

6. _____   15. _____

7. _____   16. _____

8. _____   17. _____

9. _____

GALLBLADDER AND BILE DUCTS

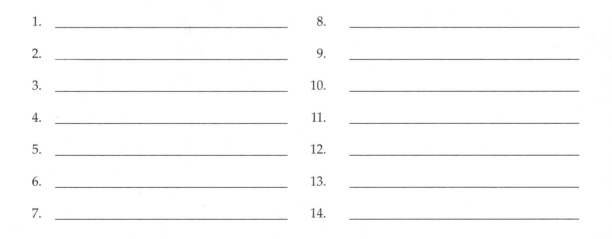

1. _____   8. _____

2. _____   9. _____

3. _____   10. _____

4. _____   11. _____

5. _____   12. _____

6. _____   13. _____

7. _____   14. _____

THE SMALL INTESTINE

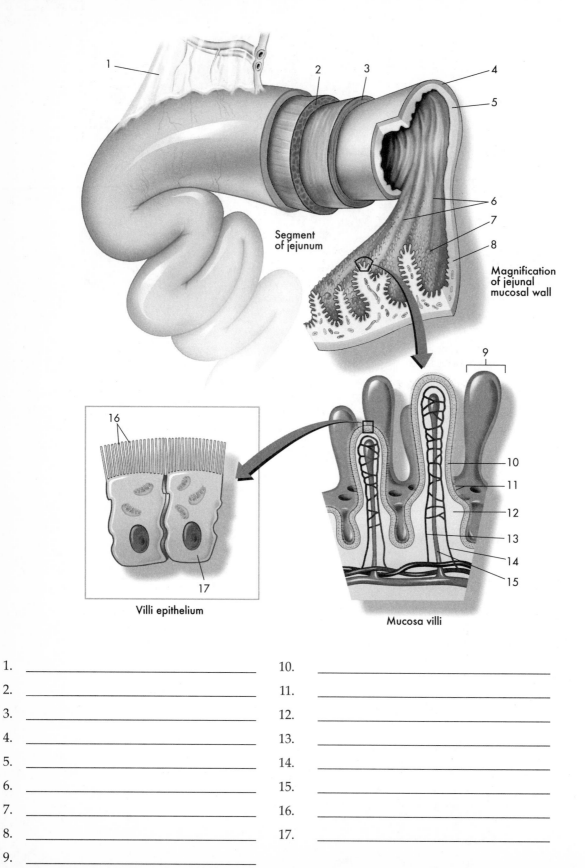

Segment of jejunum

Magnification of jejunal mucosal wall

Villi epithelium

Mucosa villi

1. _____

2. _____

3. _____

4. _____

5. _____

6. _____

7. _____

8. _____

9. _____

10. _____

11. _____

12. _____

13. _____

14. _____

15. _____

16. _____

17. _____

THE LARGE INTESTINE

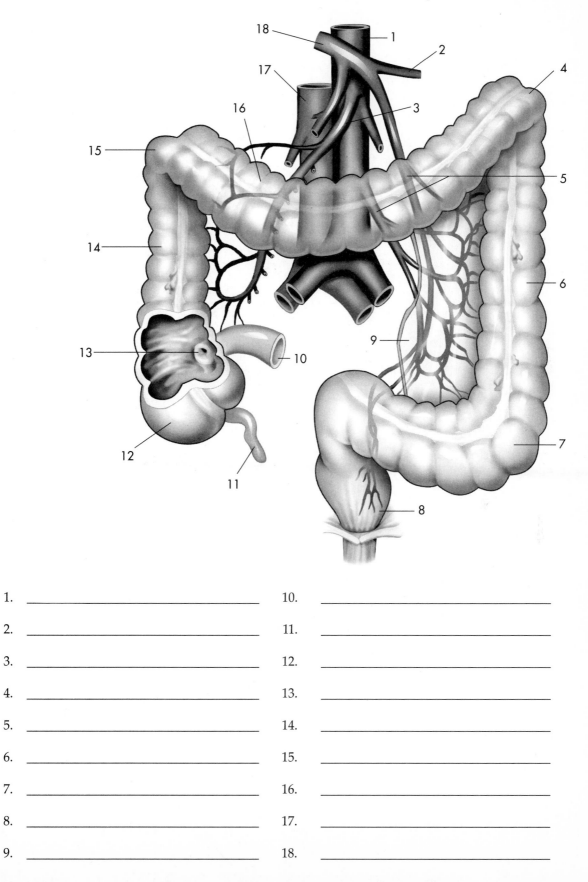

1. _____   10. _____

2. _____   11. _____

3. _____   12. _____

4. _____   13. _____

5. _____   14. _____

6. _____   15. _____

7. _____   16. _____

8. _____   17. _____

9. _____   18. _____

Nutrition and Metabolism

Most of us love to eat, but do the foods we enjoy provide us with the basic food types necessary for good nutrition? The body, a finely tuned machine, requires a balance of carbohydrates, fats, proteins, vitamins, and minerals to function properly. These nutrients must be digested, absorbed, and circulated to cells constantly to accommodate the numerous activities that occur throughout the body. The use the body makes of foods once these processes are completed is called *metabolism*.

The liver plays a major role in the metabolism of food. It helps maintain a normal blood glucose level, removes toxins from the blood, processes blood immediately after it leaves the gastrointestinal tract, and initiates the first steps of protein and fat metabolism.

This chapter also discusses basal metabolic rate (BMR). The BMR is the rate at which food is catabolized under basal conditions. This test and the protein-bound iodine (PBI) are indirect measures of thyroid gland functioning. The total metabolic rate (TMR) is the amount of energy, expressed in calories, used by the body each day.

Finally, maintaining a constant body temperature is a function of the hypothalamus and a challenge for the metabolic factors of the body. Review of this chapter is necessary to provide you with an understanding of the "fuel" (nutrition) necessary to maintain this complex homeostatic machine—the body.

TOPICS FOR REVIEW

Before progressing to Chapter 19, you should be able to define and contrast catabolism and anabolism. Your review should include the metabolic roles of carbohydrates, fats, proteins, vitamins, and minerals. Your study should conclude with an understanding of the basal metabolic rate, physiological mechanisms that regulate body temperature, and the common metabolic and eating disorders.

THE ROLE OF THE LIVER

Fill in the blanks.

The liver plays an important role in the mechanical digestion of lipids because it secretes
(1) _____. It also produces two of the plasma proteins that play an essential role in blood clotting. These two proteins are (2) _____ and
(3) _____. Additionally, liver cells store several substances, notably vitamins A and D and (4) _____. Finally, the liver is assisted by a unique structural feature of the blood vessels that supply it. This arrangement, known as the
(5) _____ _____
_____ , allows toxins to be removed from the bloodstream before nutrients are distributed throughout the body.

NUTRIENT METABOLISM

Match the term with the definition. (Answers may be used more than once.)

_____ 6.	Used if cells have inadequate amounts of glucose to catabolize	A. Carbohydrate
_____ 7.	Preferred energy food	B. Fat
_____ 8.	Amino acids	C. Protein
_____ 9.	Fat soluble	D. Vitamins
_____ 10.	Required for nerve conduction	E. Minerals
_____ 11.	Glycolysis	
_____ 12.	Inorganic elements found naturally in the earth	
_____ 13.	Pyruvic acid	

Circle the word or phrase that does not belong.

14. Glycolysis	Citric acid cycle	ATP	Bile
15. Adipose	Amino acids	Triglycerides	Lipid
16. A	D	M	K
17. Iron	Proteins	Amino acids	Essential
18. Hydrocortisone	Insulin	Growth hormone	Epinephrine
19. Sodium	Calcium	Zinc	Folic acid
20. Thiamine	Niacin	Ascorbic acid	Riboflavin

▶ *If you have had difficulty with this section, review pages 566-574.*

METABOLIC RATES

Circle the correct answer.

21. The rate at which food is catabolized under basal conditions is the:

     A. TMR
     B. PBI
     C. BMR
     D. ATP

22. The total amount of energy used by the body per day is the:
     A. TMR
     B. PBI
     C. BMR
     D. ATP

23. A/an _____ is the amount of energy needed to raise the temperature of 1 gram of water 1° Celsius.
     A. Calorie
     B. Kilocalorie
     C. ATP
     D. BMR

24. Which of the following is a factor when determining the BMR?
     A. Sex
     B. Age
     C. Size
     D. All of the above

25. Which of the following is a factor when determining the TMR?
     A. Exercise
     B. Food intake
     C. Environmental temperature
     D. All of the above

▶ *If you have had difficulty with this section, review page 574.*

METABOLIC AND EATING DISORDERS

Choose the correct response.

_____ 26.	Insulin deficiency is a symptom of this disorder	A. BMR
_____ 27.	Behavioral disorder characterized by chronic refusal to eat	B. Diabetes mellitus
_____ 28.	An advanced form of PCM	C. Anorexia nervosa
_____ 29.	Results from a deficiency of calories in general and protein in particular	D. Bulimia
_____ 30.	Hypothyroidism will affect this measurement	E. Obesity
_____ 31.	Abdominal bloating	F. PCM
_____ 32.	Symptom of chronic overeating behavior	G. Marasmus
_____ 33.	Behavioral disorder characterized by insatiable craving for food alternating with periods of self-deprivation	H. Ascites

▷ *If you have had difficulty with this section, review pages 574-578.*

BODY TEMPERATURES

Circle the correct answer.

34. Over _____ of the energy released from food molecules during catabolism is converted to heat rather than being transferred to ATP.
    A. 20%
    B. 40%
    C. 60%
    D. 80%

35. Maintaining thermoregulation is a function of the:
    A. Thalamus
    B. Hypothalamus
    C. Thyroid
    D. Parathyroids

36. Transfer of heat energy to the skin, then the external environment is known as:
    A. Radiation
    B. Conduction
    C. Convection
    D. Evaporation

37. A flow of heat waves away from the blood is known as:
    A. Radiation
    B. Conduction
    C. Convection
    D. Evaporation

38. A transfer of heat energy to air that is continually flowing away from the skin is known as:
    A. Radiation
    B. Conduction
    C. Convection
    D. Evaporation

39. Heat that is absorbed by the process of water vaporization is called:
    A. Radiation
    B. Conduction
    C. Convection
    D. Evaporation

▷ *If you have had difficulty with this section, review pages 578-579.*

ABNORMAL BODY TEMPERATURE

If the statement is true, write "T" in the answer blank. If the statement is false, correct the statement by circling the incorrect term and inserting the correct term in the answer blank.

_____ 40. Pyrogens cause the thermostatic control centers of the hypothalamus to produce a fever.

_____ 41. Malignant hyperthermia is the inability to maintain a normal body temperature in extremely cold environments.

_____ 42. Frostbite is local damage to tissues caused by extremely low temperatures.

_____ 43. Heat exhaustion is characterized by body temperatures of 41° Celsius or higher.

_____ 44. Dantrium is used to prevent or relieve the effects of frostbite.

▷ *If you have had difficulty with this section, review pages 579-581.*

UNSCRAMBLE THE WORDS

45. **L R I E V**

46. **T A O B A L I C M S**

47. **O M N I A**

48. **Y P U R C V I**

Take the circled letters, unscramble them, and fill in the statement.

How the magician paid his bills.

49.

APPLYING WHAT YOU KNOW

50. Dr. Carey was concerned about Deborrah. Her daily food intake provided fewer calories than her TMR. If this trend continues, what will be the result? If it continues over a long period of time, what eating disorder might Deborrah develop?

51. Kathryn Arce was experiencing fatigue and a blood test revealed that she was slightly anemic. What mineral will her doctor most likely prescribe? What dietary sources might you suggest that she emphasize in her daily intake?

52. Mr. Mobley was training daily for an upcoming marathon. Three days before the 25 mile event, he suddenly quit his daily routine of jogging and switched to a diet high in carbohydrates. Why did Mr. Mobley suddenly switch his routine of training?

53. Word Find

Can you find the 18 terms from this chapter that are listed below? Words may be spelled top to bottom, bottom to top, right to left, left to right, or diagonally.

```
C  C  C  B  W  E  F  F  L  J  V  G  G  S
A  T  N  L  W  E  U  O  Z  I  E  L  I  B
R  K  K  P  Z  F  R  I  T  P  O  Y  K  L
B  Q  M  I  N  E  R  A  L  S  J  C  C  P
O  S  S  N  C  X  M  I  D  B  D  O  W  P
H  S  I  Y  O  I  T  X  H  I  N  L  S  N
Y  E  L  N  N  I  K  W  W  D  S  Y  N  S
D  G  O  S  O  W  T  I  U  E  H  S  C  N
R  M  B  Y  T  I  W  C  Z  N  N  I  A  A
A  R  A  Q  W  A  T  B  E  I  G  S  J  M
T  E  T  F  N  I  F  A  E  V  E  W  T  Y
E  V  A  P  O  R  A  T  I  O  N  D  T  E
S  I  C  N  E  S  O  P  I  D  A  O  F  E
H  L  Y  K  I  R  E  B  V  P  A  H  C  J
I  W  E  E  P  A  D  F  T  E  A  R  G  G
```

ATP	Conduction	Liver
Adipose	Convection	Minerals
BMR	Evaporation	Proteins
Bile	Fats	Radiation
Carbohydrates	Glycerol	TMR
Catabolism	Glycolysis	Vitamins

DID YOU KNOW?

The amount of energy required for a person to raise a 200-pound man 15 feet in the air is about the amount of energy in one large calorie.

NUTRITION/METABOLISM

Fill in the crossword puzzle.

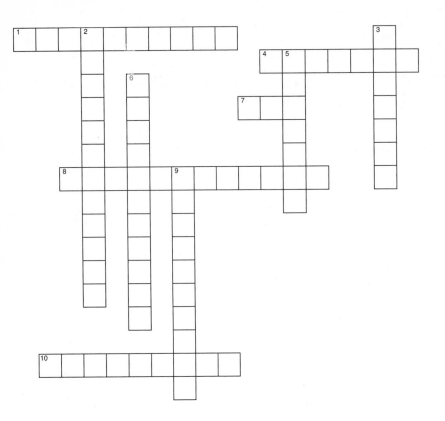

ACROSS

1. Breaks food molecules down releasing stored energy
4. Amount of energy needed to raise the temperature of one gram of water 1° Celsius
7. Rate of metabolism when a person is lying down, but awake (abbreviation)
8. A series of reactions that join glucose molecules together to form glycogen
10. Builds food molecules into complex substances

DOWN

2. Occurs when food molecules enter cells and undergo many chemical changes there
3. Organic molecule needed in small quantities for normal metabolism throughout the body
5. Oxygen-using
6. A unit of measure for heat, also known as a large calorie
9. Takes place in the cytoplasm of a cell and changes glucose to pyruvic acid

CHECK YOUR KNOWLEDGE

Multiple Choice

Circle the correct answer.

1. What is the process by which pyruvic acid is broken down into carbon dioxide called?
   A. Glycogenesis
   B. Citric acid cycle
   C. Glycolysis
   D. Pyruvic acid cycle

2. The anabolism of glucose produces which of the following?
   A. Glycogen
   B. Amino acid
   C. Rennin
   D. Starch

3. Which of the following is a major hormone in the body that aids carbohydrate metabolism?
   A. Oxytocin
   B. Epinephrine
   C. Insulin
   D. Growth hormone

4. The total metabolic rate is which of the following?
   A. The amount of fats we consume in a 24-hour period
   B. The same as the BMR
   C. The amount of energy expressed in calories used by the body per day
   D. Cannot be calculated

5. When your consumption of calories equals your TMR, your weight will do which of the following?
   A. Increase
   B. Remain the same
   C. Fluctuate
   D. Decrease

6. Which of the following is a normal glucose level?
   A. 40 to 80 mg/100 ml blood
   B. 80 to 120 mg/100 ml blood
   C. 100 to 140 mg/100 ml blood
   D. 180 to 220 mg/100 ml blood

7. When glucose is *not* available, the body will next catabolize which of the following energy sources?
   A. Fats
   B. Proteins
   C. Minerals
   D. Vitamins

8. Maintaining the homeostasis of the body temperature is the responsibility of which of the following?
   A. Hypothalamus
   B. Environmental condition in which we live
   C. Circulatory system
   D. None of the above

9. The liver plays an important role in the mechanical digestion of lipids because it secretes:
   A. Glucose molecules
   B. Bile
   C. Glycogen
   D. Citric acid

10. What is the primary molecule the body usually breaks down as an energy source?
    A. Amino acid
    B. Pepsin
    C. Maltose
    D. Glucose

Completion

Complete the following statements using the terms listed below. (Some words may be used more than once.)

A. Vitamins
B. Insulin
C. Carbohydrates
D. Fats
E. Glycolysis
F. Heat

G. ATP
H. Sodium
I. Proteins
J. Citric acid cycle
K. Calcium
L. Glycogen loading

11. Proper nutrition requires the balance of the three basic food types: _____, _____, and _____.

12. The process that changes glucose to pyruvic acid is called _____.

13. Once glucose has been changed to pyruvic acid, another process in which pyruvic acid is changed to carbon dioxide takes place. This reaction is known as the _____.

14. A direct source of energy for doing cellular work is _____.

15. The only hormone that lowers blood glucose level is _____.

16. When cells have an inadequate amount of glucose to catabolize they will catabolize _____.

17. Some athletes consume large amounts of carbohydrates 2 to 3 days before an athletic event to store glycogen in skeletal muscles. This practice is called _____.

18. Organic molecules needed in small amounts for normal metabolism are _____.

19. Two minerals necessary for nerve conduction and contraction of muscle fibers are _____ and _____.

20. During catabolism, food molecules are converted to _____ rather than being transported to ATP.

CHAPTER 19

The Urinary System

Living produces wastes. Wherever people live, work, or play, wastes accumulate. To keep these areas healthy, there must be a method of disposing of these wastes such as a sanitation department. Wastes also accumulate in your body. The conversion of food and gases into substances and energy necessary for survival results in waste products. A large percentage of these wastes is removed by the urinary system.

Two vital organs, the kidneys, cleanse the blood of the many waste products that are continually produced as a result of the metabolism of food in the body cells. They eliminate these wastes in the form of urine.

Urine formation is the result of three processes: filtration, reabsorption, and secretion. These processes occur in successive portions of the microscopic units of the kidneys known as *nephrons*. The amount of urine produced by the nephrons is controlled primarily by the hormones ADH and aldosterone.

After urine is produced, it is drained from the renal pelvis by the ureters to flow into the bladder. The bladder then stores the urine until it is voided through the urethra.

If waste products are allowed to accumulate in the body, they soon become poisonous, a condition called *uremia*. A knowledge of the urinary system is necessary to understand how the body rids itself of waste and avoids toxicity.

TOPICS FOR REVIEW

Before progressing to Chapter 20, you should have an understanding of the structure and function of the organs of the urinary system. Your review should include knowledge of the nephron and its role in urine production. Your study should conclude with a review of the three main processes involved in urine production, the mechanisms that control urine volume, and the major renal and urinary disorders.

KIDNEYS

FORMATION OF URINE

Circle the correct answer.

1. The outermost portion of the kidney is known as the:
   A. Medulla
   B. Papilla
   C. Pelvis
   D. Pyramid
   E. Cortex

2. The saclike structure that surrounds the glomerulus is the:
   A. Renal pelvis
   B. Calyx
   C. Bowman's capsule
   D. Cortex
   E. None of the above

3. The renal corpuscle is made up of the:
   A. Bowman's capsule and proximal convoluted tubule
   B. Glomerulus and proximal convoluted tubule
   C. Bowman's capsule and the distal convoluted tubule
   D. Glomerulus and the distal convoluted tubule
   E. Bowman's capsule and the glomerulus

4. Which of the following functions is *not* performed by the kidneys?
   A. Help maintain homeostasis
   B. Remove wastes from the blood
   C. Produce ADH
   D. Remove electrolytes from the blood

5. _____ % of the glomerular filtrate is reabsorbed.
   A. 20
   B. 40
   C. 75
   D. 85
   E. 99

6. The glomerular filtration rate is _____ ml per minute.
   A. 1.25
   B. 12.5
   C. 125.0
   D. 1250.0
   E. None of the above

7. Glucose reabsorption begins in the:
   A. Loop of Henle
   B. Proximal convoluted tubule
   C. Distal convoluted tubule
   D. Glomerulus
   E. None of the above

8. Reabsorption does *not* occur in the:
   A. Loop of Henle
   B. Proximal convoluted tubule
   C. Distal convoluted tubule
   D. Collecting tubules
   E. Calyx

9. The greater the amount of salt intake, the:
   A. Less salt is excreted in the urine
   B. More salt is reabsorbed
   C. The more salt is excreted in the urine
   D. None of the above

10. Which one of the following substances is secreted by diffusion?
    A. Sodium ions
    B. Certain drugs
    C. Ammonia
    D. Hydrogen ions
    E. Potassium ions

11. Which of the following statements about ADH is *not* correct?
    A. It is stored by the pituitary gland.
    B. It makes the collecting tubules less permeable to water.
    C. It makes the distal convoluted tubules more permeable.
    D. It is produced by the hypothalamus.

12. Which of the following statements about aldosterone is *not* correct?
    A. It is secreted by the adrenal cortex.
    B. It is a water-retaining hormone.
    C. It is a salt-retaining hormone.
    D. All of the above are correct.

Choose the correct term and write the letter in the space next to the appropriate definition below.

_____ 13.	Functioning unit of the urinary system	A. Medulla
_____ 14.	Abnormal characteristic of urine	B. Cortex
_____ 15.	Normal characteristic of urine	C. Pyramids
_____ 16.	Outer part of the kidney	D. Papilla
_____ 17.	Together with Bowman's capsule forms the renal corpuscle	E. Pelvis
_____ 18.	Division of the renal pelvis	F. Calyx
_____ 19.	Cup-shaped top of a nephron	G. Nephrons
_____ 20.	Innermost end of a pyramid	H. Creatinine
_____ 21.	Extension of the proximal tubule	I. Albumin
_____ 22.	Triangular-shaped divisions of the medulla of the kidney	J. Bowman's capsule
_____ 23.	An expansion of the upper end of a ureter	K. Glomerulus
_____ 24.	Inner portion of the kidney	L. Loop of Henle

▶ *If you have had difficulty with this section, review pages 588-598.*

URETERS
URINARY BLADDER
URETHRA

Indicate which organ is identified by the following descriptions by inserting the appropriate letter in the answer blank.

A. Ureters   B. Bladder   C. Urethra

_____ 25. Between urinary meatus and bladder

_____ 26. Rugae

_____ 27. Lowest part of the urinary tract

_____ 28. Lining membrane richly supplied with sensory nerve endings

_____ 29. Lies behind the pubic symphysis

_____ 30. Dual function in the male

_____ 31. 1 1/2 inches long in the female

_____ 32. Drain the renal pelvis

_____ 33. Surrounded by the prostate in the male

_____ 34. Elastic fibers and involuntary muscle fibers

_____ 35. 10 to 12 inches long

_____ 36. Trigone

Fill in the blanks.

37. The physical, chemical, and microscopic examination of urine is termed

    _____.

38. The urinary tract is lined with _____ _____.

39. Urine specimens are often spun in a _____ to force suspended particles
    to the bottom of a test tube.

40. The absence of urine is known as _____.

41. Clinical studies have proven that improper catheterization techniques cause
    _____ in hospitalized patients.

42. In the male, the urethra serves a dual function: a passageway for urine and

    _____.

43. The external opening of the urethra is the _____

    _____.

▷ *If you have had difficulty with this section, review pages 598-601.*

MICTURITION

Fill in the blanks.

The terms (44) _____, (45) _____, and
(46) _____ all refer to the passage of urine from the body or the emptying
of the bladder. The sphincters guard the bladder. The (47) _____

_____ _____ is the sphincter located at
the bladder (48) _____ and is involuntary. The external urethral sphincter
encircles the (49) _____ and is under
(50) _____ control. As the bladder fills, nervous impulses are transmitted to
the spinal cord and an (51) _____ is initiated. Urine then enters the
(52) _____ to be eliminated. Urinary
(53) _____ is a condition in which no urine is voided. Urinary
(54) _____ is when the kidneys do not produce any urine, but the bladder
retains its ability to empty itself. The term (55) _____

_____ is often used to describe the type of urine loss associated with laugh-
ing, coughing, or heavy lifting.

▷ *If you have had difficulty with this section, review pages 600-601.*

RENAL AND URINARY DISORDERS

Select the correct disorder from the clues that are provided.

_____ 56.	Urine backs up into the kidneys causing swelling of the renal pelvis and calyces	A. Pyelonephritis
_____ 57.	Kidney stones	B. Renal colic
_____ 58.	Intermittent dribbling of urine	C. Renal calculi
_____ 59.	Blood in the urine	D. Acute glomerulonephritis
_____ 60.	Inflammation of the bladder	E. Proteinuria
_____ 61.	Inflammation of the renal pelvis and connective tissues of the kidney	F. Hematuria
_____ 62.	An abrupt reduction in kidney function characterized by oliguria and a sharp rise in nitrogenous compounds in the blood	G. Overflow incontinence
_____ 63.	Progressive condition resulting from gradual loss of nephrons	H. Acute renal failure
_____ 64.	Intense kidney pain caused by obstruction of the ureters by large kidney stones	I. Hydronephrosis
_____ 65.	Most common form of kidney disease caused by a delayed immune response to streptococcal infection	J. Chronic renal failure
_____ 66.	Albumin in the urine	K. Cystitis
_____ 67.	Inflammation of the urethra that commonly results from bacterial infection	L. Urethritis

▶ *If you have had difficulty with this section, review pages 601-609.*

UNSCRAMBLE THE WORDS

68. A Y X L C

69. G V N O I D I

70. A L P A L I P

71. S G U L L O U M R E

Take the circled letters, unscramble them, and fill in the statement.

What Betty saw while cruising down the Nile.

72.

APPLYING WHAT YOU KNOW

73. John suffered from low levels of ADH. What primary urinary symptom would he notice?
74. Bud was in a diving accident and his spinal cord was severed. He was paralyzed from the waist down and as a result was incontinent. His physician, Dr. Welch, was concerned about the continuous residual urine buildup. What was the reason for concern?
75. Mrs. Lynch had a prolonged surgical procedure and experienced problems with urinary retention postoperatively. A urinary catheter was inserted into her bladder for the elimination of urine. Several days later Mrs. Lynch developed cystitis. What might be a possible cause of this diagnosis?
76. Mr. Dietz, an accident victim, was admitted to the hospital several hours ago. His chart indicates that he had been hemorrhaging at the scene of the accident. Nurse Petersen has been closely monitoring his urinary output and has noted that it has dropped to 10 ml/hr. (The normal urine output for a healthy adult is approximately 30 to 60 ml/hr.) What might explain this drop in urine output?

77. Word Find

Can you find the 18 terms from this chapter that are listed below? Words may be spelled top to bottom, bottom to top, right to left, left to right, or diagonally.

```
H N O I T I R U T C I M N M Y
V E Q N G A L L I P A P S E S
T P M C O L D U J Y S I N D D
L H G O X I O W C G V D I U J
C R F N D B T M T L I M B K L
P O O T X I C A E K A P X L D
Q N U I E G A P R R T C W A O
B J R N T T L Y T U Y G D M
S D E E R G Y P Y V L L P H Z
I H T N O U X W D S X I U J G
M X E C C Y S T I T I S F S Q
J O R E D D A L B U E S G B S
Y I S E B V L L B H V Q L U L
```

ADH
Bladder
Calculi
Calyx
Cortex
Cystitis
Filtration
Glomerulus
Hemodialysis
Incontinence
Kidney
Medulla
Micturition
Nephron
Papilla
Pelvis
Pyramids
Ureters

DID YOU KNOW?

If the tubules in a kidney were stretched out and untangled, there would be 70 miles of them.

One out of every eight men will develop prostate cancer in his lifetime.

URINARY SYSTEM

Fill in the crossword puzzle.

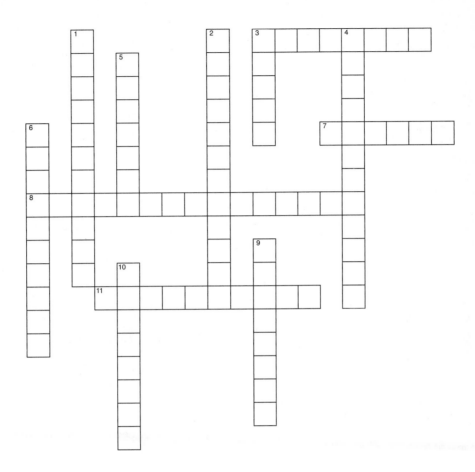

ACROSS

3. Bladder infection
7. Absence of urine
8. Passage of a tube into the bladder to withdraw urine
11. Network of blood capillaries tucked into Bowman's capsule

DOWN

1. Urination
2. Ultrasound generator used to break up kidney stones
3. Division of the renal pelvis
4. Voiding involuntarily
5. Area on posterior bladder wall free of rugae
6. Glucose in the urine
9. Large amount of urine
10. Scanty urine

CHECK YOUR KNOWLEDGE

Multiple Choice

Circle the correct answer.

1. Which of the following is true of urinary catheterization?
   A. It can be used to treat retention.
   B. It requires aseptic technique.
   C. It can lead to cystitis.
   D. All of the above are true.

2. Which of the following processes are used by the artificial kidney to remove waste materials from blood?
   A. Pinocytosis
   B. Dialysis
   C. Catheterization
   D. Active transport

3. Failure of the kidneys to remove wastes from the blood will result in which of the following?
   A. Retention
   B. Anuria
   C. Incontinence
   D. Uremia

4. Hydrogen ions are transferred from blood into the urine during which of the following processes?
   A. Secretion
   B. Filtration
   C. Reabsorption
   D. All of the above

5. Which of the following conditions would be considered normal in an infant under 2 years of age?
   A. Retention
   B. Cystitis
   C. Incontinence
   D. Anuria

6. Which of the following steps involved in urine formation allows the blood to retain most body nutrients?
   A. Secretion
   B. Filtration
   C. Reabsorption
   D. All of the above

7. Voluntary control of micturition is achieved by the action of which of the following?
   A. Internal urethral sphincter
   B. External urethral sphincter
   C. Trigone
   D. Bladder muscles

8. What is the structure that carries urine from the kidney to the bladder called?
   A. Urethra
   B. Bowman's capsule
   C. Ureter
   D. Renal pelvis

9. What are the capillary loops contained within Bowman's capsule called?
   A. Convoluted tubules
   B. Glomeruli
   C. Limbs of Henle's loop
   D. Collecting ducts

10. The triangular divisions of the medulla of the kidney are known as:
    A. Pyramids
    B. Papillae
    C. Calyces
    D. Nephrons

Matching

Select the correct answer from column B for each item in column A. (Only one answer is correct.)

Column A

_____ 11. Retention

_____ 12. Anuria

_____ 13. Cystitis

_____ 14. Micturition

_____ 15. Oliguria

_____ 16. Polyuria

_____ 17. Incontinence

_____ 18. Hematuria

_____ 19. Suppression

_____ 20. Reabsorption

Column B

A. Involuntary voiding

B. Movement of substance out of renal tubules into blood

C. Absence of urine

D. Urination

E. Bladder does not empty

F. Inflammation of the urinary bladder

G. Traces of blood in the urine

H. Large amount of urine

I. Kidneys not producing urine

J. Scanty amount of urine

URINARY SYSTEM

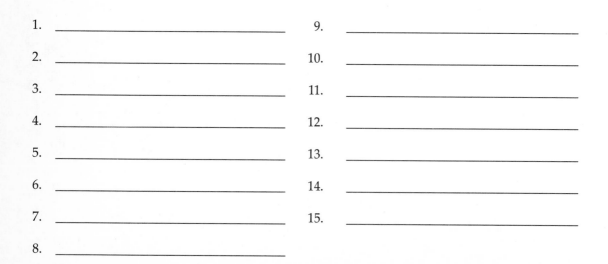

1. _____   9. _____

2. _____   10. _____

3. _____   11. _____

4. _____   12. _____

5. _____   13. _____

6. _____   14. _____

7. _____   15. _____

8. _____

KIDNEY

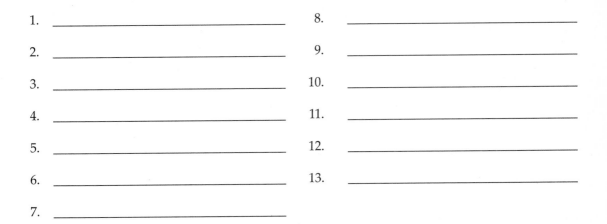

1. _____   8. _____

2. _____   9. _____

3. _____   10. _____

4. _____   11. _____

5. _____   12. _____

6. _____   13. _____

7. _____

NEPHRON

1. _____

2. _____

3. _____

4. _____

5. _____

6. _____

7. _____

8. _____

9. _____

10. _____

11. _____

12. _____

13. _____

Fluid and Electrolyte Balance

Referring to the first chapter in your text, you will recall that survival depends on the body's ability to maintain or restore homeostasis. Specifically, *homeostasis* means that the body fluids remain constant within very narrow limits. These fluids are classified as either intracellular fluid (ICF) or extracellular fluid (ECF). As their names imply, intracellular fluid lies within the cells and extracellular fluid is located outside the cells. A balance between these two fluids is maintained by certain body mechanisms. They are: 1) the adjustment of fluid output to fluid intake under normal circumstances; 2) the concentration of electrolytes in the extracellular fluid; 3) the capillary blood pressure; and finally, 4) the concentration of proteins in the blood.

Comprehension of how these mechanisms maintain and restore fluid balance is necessary for an understanding of the complexities of homeostasis and its relationship to the survival of the individual.

TOPICS FOR REVIEW

Before progressing to Chapter 21, you should review the types of body fluids and their subdivisions. Your study should include the mechanisms that maintain fluid balance and the nature and importance of electrolytes in body fluids. You should be able to give examples of common fluid imbalances, and have an understanding of the role of fluid and electrolyte balance in the maintenance of homeostasis.

BODY FLUIDS

Circle the correct answer.

1. The largest volume of water by far lies (inside or outside) cells.
2. Interstitial fluid is (intracellular or extracellular).
3. Plasma is (intracellular or extracellular).
4. Obese people have a (lower or higher) water content per pound of body weight than thin people.
5. Infants have (more or less) water in comparison to body weight than adults of either sex.
6. There is a rapid (increase or decline) in the proportion of body water to body weight during the first year of life.
7. The female body contains slightly (more or less) water per pound of weight.
8. In general, as age increases, the amount of water per pound of body weight (increases or decreases).
9. Excluding adipose tissue, approximately (55% or 85%) of body weight is water.
10. The term (fluid balance or fluid compartments) means the volumes of ICF, IF, plasma, and the total volume of water in the body all remain relatively constant.

▷ *If you have had difficulty with this section, review pages 616-626.*

MECHANISMS THAT MAINTAIN FLUID BALANCE

Circle the correct answer.

11. Which one of the following is *not* a positively charged ion?
    A. Chloride
    B. Calcium
    C. Sodium
    D. Potassium

12. Which one of the following is *not* a negatively charged ion?
    A. Chloride
    B. Bicarbonate
    C. Phosphate
    D. Sodium

13. The most abundant electrolyte in blood plasma is:
    A. NaCl
    B. KMg
    C. HCO_3
    D. HPO_4
    E. $CaPO_4$

14. The smallest amount of water comes from:
    A. Water in foods that are eaten
    B. Ingested liquids
    C. Water formed from catabolism
    D. None of the above

15. The greatest amount of water lost from the body is from the:
    A. Lungs
    B. Skin by diffusion
    C. Skin by sweat
    D. Feces
    E. Kidneys

16. Which one of the following is *not* a major factor that influences extracellular and intracellular fluid volumes?
    A. The concentration of electrolytes in the extracellular fluid
    B. The capillary blood pressure
    C. The concentration of proteins in blood
    D. All of the above are important factors

17. The type of fluid output that changes the most is:
    A. Water loss in the feces
    B. Water loss from the skin
    C. Water loss via the lungs
    D. Water loss in the urine
    E. None of the above

18. The chief regulators of sodium within the body are the:
    A. Lungs
    B. Sweat glands
    C. Kidneys
    D. Large intestine
    E. None of the above

19. Which of the following is *not* correct?
    A. Fluid output must equal fluid intake.
    B. ADH controls salt reabsorption in the kidney.
    C. Water follows sodium.
    D. Renal tubule regulation of salt and water is the most important factor in determining urine volume.
    E. All of the above are correct.

20. Diuretics work on all but which one of the following?
    A. Proximal tubule
    B. Loop of Henle
    C. Distal tubule
    D. Collecting ducts
    E. Diuretics work on all of the above

21. Of all the sodium-containing secretions, the one with the largest volume is:
    A. Saliva
    B. Gastric secretions
    C. Bile
    D. Pancreatic juice
    E. Intestinal secretions

22. The higher the capillary blood pressure, the _____ the amount of interstitial fluid.
    A. Smaller
    B. Larger
    C. There is no relationship between capillary blood pressure and volume of interstitial fluid

23. An increase in capillary blood pressure will lead to _____ in blood volume.
    A. An increase
    B. A decrease
    C. No change
    D. None of the above

24. Which one of the fluid compartments varies the most in volume?
    A. Intracellular
    B. Interstitial
    C. Extracellular
    D. Plasma

If the statement is true, write "T" in the answer blank. If the statement is false, correct the statement by circling the incorrect term and inserting the correct term in the answer blank.

_____ 25. The three sources of fluid intake are the liquids we drink, the foods we eat, and water formed by the anabolism of foods.

_____ 26. The body maintains fluid balance mainly by changing the volume of urine excreted to match changes in the volume of fluid intake.

_____ 27. Some output of fluid will occur as long as life continues.

_____ 28. Glucose is an example of an electrolyte.

_____ 29. Where sodium goes, water soon follows.

_____ 30. Excess aldosterone leads to hypovolemia.

_____ 31. Diuretics have their effect on glomerular function.

_____ 32. Typical daily intake and output totals should be approximately 1200 ml.

_____ 33. Bile is a sodium-containing internal secretion.

_____ 34. The average daily diet contains about 500 mEq of sodium.

▶ *If you have had difficulty with this section, review pages 620-626.*

FLUID IMBALANCES

Fill in the blanks.

(35) _____ is the fluid imbalance seen most often. In this condition, interstitial fluid volume (36) _____ first, but eventually, if treatment has not been given, intracellular fluid and plasma volumes (37) _____.

(38) _____ can also occur, but is much less common. Giving (39) _____ _____ too rapidly or in too large amounts can put too heavy a burden on the (40) _____.

(41) _____ describes a blood sodium level above 145 mEq/L.

(42) _____ is a clinical term used to describe blood potassium levels above 5.1 mEq/L.

▶ *If you have had difficulty with this section, review pages 626-628.*

APPLYING WHAT YOU KNOW

43. Mrs. Titus was asked to keep an accurate record of her fluid intake and output. She was concerned because the two did not balance. What is a possible explanation for this?

44. Nurse Briker was caring for a patient who was receiving diuretics. What special nursing implications should be followed for patients on this therapy?

45. Jack Sprat was 6'5" and weighed 185 lbs. His wife was 5'6" and weighed 185 lbs. Whose body contained more water?

46.   Word Find

Can you find the 12 terms from this chapter that are listed below? Words may be spelled top to bottom, bottom to top, right to left, left to right, or diagonally.

```
S  T  V  H  O  M  E  O  S  T  A  S  I  S  H
I  E  D  E  M  A  S  Q  A  L  P  U  E  G  L
M  M  L  U  F  L  U  I  D  O  Y  O  I  S  L
W  S  B  E  A  E  C  O  L  D  P  N  I  E  R
L  I  T  A  C  V  S  H  Q  O  C  E  H  B  C
L  L  X  J  L  T  E  A  W  Y  B  V  Q  Q  O
I  O  O  P  E  A  R  U  C  T  C  A  A  R  I
N  B  H  R  X  S  N  O  I  I  P  R  T  C  N
S  A  O  X  M  G  J  C  L  N  J  T  B  A  H
I  N  X  X  D  V  U  D  E  Y  K  N  Y  O  C
E  A  A  J  Q  D  I  U  R  E  T  I  C  S  X
I  F  C  J  A  M  P  V  E  N  B  E  Y  F  W
V  F  K  T  Q  X  R  M  D  D  S  I  V  O  T
E  T  T  Z  N  T  R  P  X  I  M  L  J  F  I
S  W  Y  A  P  V  Q  N  S  K  T  K  W  B  P
```

Aldosterone	Edema	Imbalance
Anabolism	Electrolyte	Intravenous
Catabolism	Fluid	Ions
Diuretics	Homeostasis	Kidney

DID YOU KNOW?

The best fluid replacement drink is to add 1/4 tsp. of table salt to one quart of water.

FLUID/ELECTROLYTES

Fill in the crossword puzzle.

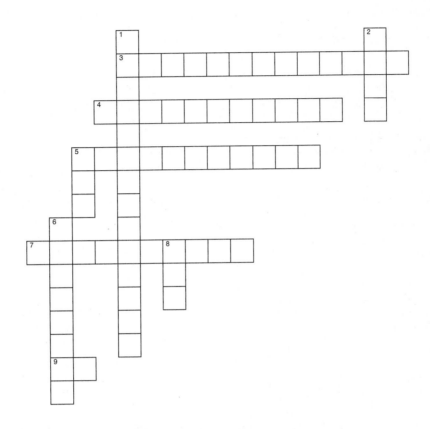

ACROSS

3. Result of rapidly given intravenous fluids
4. Result of large loss of body fluids
5. Compound that dissociates in solution into ions
7. To break up
9. A subdivision of extracellular fluid (abbreviation)

DOWN

1. Organic substance that doesn't dissociate in solution
2. Dissociated particles of an electrolyte that carry an electrical charge
5. Fluid outside cells (abbreviation)
6. "Causing urine"
8. Fluid inside cells (abbreviation)

CHECK YOUR KNOWLEDGE

Multiple Choice

Circle the correct answer.

1. Which of the following statements, if any, is *false*?
   A. The more fat present in the body, the more total water content per unit of weight.
   B. Infants have more water in comparison with body weight than adults.
   C. As age increases, the amount of water per pound of body weight decreases.
   D. All of the above statements are true.

2. Avenues of fluid output include which of the following?
   A. Skin
   B. Lungs
   C. Kidneys
   D. All of the above

3. Excessive water loss and fluid imbalance can result from which of the following?
   A. Diarrhea
   B. Vomiting
   C. Severe burns
   D. All of the above

4. What factor is primarily responsible for moving water from interstitial fluid into blood?
   A. Aldosterone secretions
   B. Pressure in blood capillaries
   C. Protein concentration of blood plasma
   D. Antidiuretic hormone secretions

5. What is the chief regulator of sodium levels in body fluids?
   A. Kidney
   B. Intestine
   C. Blood
   D. Lung

6. If blood sodium concentration decreases, what does blood volume do?
   A. Increases
   B. Decreases
   C. Remains the same
   D. None of the above

7. Which of the following is true of body water?
   A. It is obtained from the liquids we drink.
   B. It is obtained from the foods we eat.
   C. It is formed by the catabolism of food.
   D. All of the above are true.

8. Edema may result from which of the following?
   A. Retention of electrolytes
   B. Decreased blood pressure
   C. Increased concentration of blood plasma proteins
   D. All of the above

9. The most abundant and most important positive plasma ion is which of the following?
   A. Sodium
   B. Chloride
   C. Calcium
   D. Oxygen

10. Which of the following is true when extracellular fluid volume decreases?
    A. Aldosterone secretion increases.
    B. Kidney tubule reabsorption of sodium increases.
    C. Urine volume decreases.
    D. All of the above are true.

Completion

Complete the following statements using the terms listed below.

A. Aldosterone
B. Edema
C. Proteins
D. Decreases
E. Diuretic

F. Electrolytes
G. Positive
H. Antidiuretic hormone
I. Dehydration
J. Extracellular fluid

K. Plasma
L. Urine
M. Interstitial fluid
N. Fluid balance

11. Any drug that promotes or stimulates the production of urine is called a _____.

12. The presence of abnormally large amounts of fluid in the intercellular tissue spaces of the body is called _____.

13. Water located outside of cells is called _____. It can be divided into two categories. If located in the spaces between the cells, it is called _____; and if located in blood vessels, it is called _____.

14. Compounds like sodium chloride that form ions when placed in solution are called _____.

15. When the adrenal cortex increases its secretion of aldosterone, urine volume _____.

16. Most fluids leave the body in the form of _____.

17. When fluid output is greater than fluid intake, _____ occurs.

18. How much water moves into blood from interstitial fluid depends largely on the concentration of _____ present in blood plasma. These substances act as a water-pulling or water-holding force.

19. Urine volume is regulated primarily by a hormone secreted by the posterior lobe of the pituitary gland called _____ and by a hormone secreted by the adrenal gland called _____.

20. Homeostasis of fluids is also known as _____.

CHAPTER 21

Acid-Base Balance

I t has been established in previous chapters that equilibrium between intracellular and extracellular fluid volume must exist for homeostasis. Equally important to homeostasis is the chemical acid-base balance of the body fluids. The degree of acidity or alkalinity of a body fluid is expressed in pH value. The neutral point, where a fluid would be neither acid nor alkaline, is pH 7. Increasing acidity is expressed as less than 7, and increasing alkalinity as greater than 7. Examples of body fluids that are acidic are gastric juice (1.6) and urine (6.0). Blood, on the other hand, is considered alkaline with a pH of 7.45.

Buffers are substances that prevent a sharp change in the pH of a fluid when an acid or base is added to it. They are one of several mechanisms that are constantly monitoring the pH of fluids in the body. If, for any reason, these mechanisms do not function properly, a pH imbalance occurs. These two kinds of imbalances are known as *alkalosis* and *acidosis*.

Maintaining the acid-base balance of body fluids is a matter of vital importance. If this balance varies even slightly, necessary chemical and cellular reactions cannot occur. Your review of this chapter is necessary to understand the delicate acid-base balance necessary for survival.

TOPICS FOR REVIEW

Before progressing to Chapter 22 you should have an understanding of the pH of body fluids and the mechanisms that control the pH of these fluids in the body. Your study should conclude with a review of the metabolic and respiratory types of pH imbalances.

pH OF THE BODY

Write the letter of the correct term on the blank next to the appropriate statement.

A. Acid   B. Base

_____ 1.   Lower concentration of hydrogen ions than hydroxide ions
_____ 2.   Higher concentration of hydrogen ions than hydroxide ions
_____ 3.   Gastric juice
_____ 4.   Saliva
_____ 5.   Arterial blood
_____ 6.   Venous blood
_____ 7.   Baking soda
_____ 8.   Beer
_____ 9.   Ammonia
_____ 10.   Seawater

▷ *If you have had difficulty with this section, review pages 635-636.*

MECHANISMS THAT CONTROL THE pH OF BODY FLUIDS

Circle the correct answer.

11. When carbon dioxide enters the blood, it reacts with the enzyme carbonic anhydrase to form:
    A. Sodium bicarbonate
    B. Water and carbon dioxide
    C. Ammonium chloride
    D. Bicarbonate ion
    E. Carbonic acid

12. The lungs remove _____ liters of carbonic acid each day.
    A. 10.0
    B. 15.0
    C. 20.0
    D. 25.0
    E. 30.0

13. When a buffer reacts with a strong acid, it changes the strong acid to a:
    A. Weak acid
    B. Strong base
    C. Weak base
    D. Water
    E. None of the above

14. Which one of the following is *not* a change in the blood that results from the buffering of fixed acids in tissue capillaries?
    A. The amount of carbonic acid increases slightly.
    B. The amount of bicarbonate in blood decreases.
    C. The hydrogen ion concentration of blood increases slightly.
    D. The blood pH decreases slightly.
    E. All of the above are changes that result from the buffering of fixed acids in tissue capillaries.

15. The most abundant acid in body fluids is:
    A. HCl
    B. Lactic acid
    C. Carbonic acid
    D. Acetic acid
    E. Sulfuric acid

16. The normal ratio of sodium bicarbonate to carbonic acid in arterial blood is:
    A. 5:1
    B. 10:1
    C. 15:1
    D. 20:1
    E. None of the above

17. Which of the following would *not* be a consequence of holding your breath?
    A. The amount of carbonic acid in the blood would increase.
    B. The blood pH would decrease.
    C. The body would develop an alkalosis.
    D. No carbon dioxide could leave the body.

18. The most effective regulators of blood pH are:
    A. The lungs
    B. The kidneys
    C. Buffers
    D. None of the above

19. The pH of the urine may be as low as:
    A. 1.6
    B. 2.5
    C. 3.2
    D. 4.8
    E. 7.4

20. In the distal tubule cells, the product of the reaction aided by carbonic anhydrase is:
    A. Water
    B. Carbon dioxide
    C. Water and carbon dioxide
    D. Hydrogen ions
    E. Carbonic acid

21. In the distal tubule, _____ leaves the tubule cells and enters the blood capillaries.
    A. Carbon dioxide
    B. Water
    C. HCO_3
    D. NaH_2PO_4
    E. $NaHCO_3$

If the statement is true, write "T" in the answer blank. If the statement is false, correct the statement by circling the incorrect term and inserting the correct term in the answer blank.

_____ 22. The body has three mechanisms for regulating the pH of its fluids. They are the heart mechanism, the respiratory mechanism, and the urinary mechanism.

_____ 23. Buffers consist of two kinds of substances and therefore are often called *duobuffers*.

_____ 24. Black coffee and cola are acidic on the pH scale.

_____ 25. Some athletes have adopted a technique called *bicarbonate loading*, ingesting large amounts of sodium bicarbonate ($NaHCO_3$) to counteract the effects of lactic acid buildup.

_____ 26. Anything that causes an excessive increase in respiration will, in time, produce acidosis.

_____ 27. Venous blood has a higher pH than arterial blood.

_____ 28. More acids than bases are usually excreted by the kidneys because more acids than bases usually enter the blood.

_____ 29. Blood levels of sodium bicarbonate can be regulated by the lungs.

_____ 30. Blood levels of carbonic acid can be regulated by the kidneys.

▷ *If you have had difficulty with this section, review pages 636-645.*

METABOLIC AND RESPIRATORY DISTURBANCES

Write the letter of the correct term on the blank next to the appropriate definition.

_____ 31. Emesis

_____ 32. Result of untreated diabetes

_____ 33. Chloride-containing solution

_____ 34. Bicarbonate deficit

_____ 35. Occurs during emesis and may result in metabolic alkalosis

_____ 36. Bicarbonate excess

_____ 37. Rapid breathing

_____ 38. Carbonic acid excess

_____ 39. Carbonic acid deficit

_____ 40. Emetic

A. Metabolic acidosis

B. Metabolic alkalosis

C. Respiratory acidosis

D. Respiratory alkalosis

E. Vomiting

F. Normal saline

G. Uncompensated metabolic acidosis

H. Hyperventilation

I. HCl loss

J. Ipecac

▷ *If you have had difficulty with this section, review pages 643-646.*

APPLYING WHAT YOU KNOW

41. Holly was pregnant and was experiencing repeated vomiting episodes for several days. Her doctor became concerned, admitted her to the hospital, and began intravenous administrations of normal saline. How will this help Holly?

42. Cara had a minor bladder infection. She had heard that this is often the result of the urine being less acidic than necessary and that she should drink cranberry juice to correct the acid problem. She had no cranberry juice, so she decided to substitute orange juice. What was wrong with this substitution?

43. Mr. Shearer has frequent bouts of hyperacidity of the stomach. Which will assist in neutralizing the acid more promptly: milk or milk of magnesia?

44. Word Find

Can you find the 18 terms from this chapter that are listed below? Words may be spelled top to bottom, bottom to top, right to left, left to right, or diagonally.

```
S  I  S  A  T  S  O  E  M  O  H  P  R  G
E  C  N  A  L  A  B  D  I  U  L  F  E  F
T  S  Y  E  N  D  I  K  W  T  I  K  A  J
Y  D  M  N  D  E  J  W  L  P  T  D  J  I
L  D  N  O  L  H  V  W  O  U  H  D  O  I
O  V  E  R  H  Y  D  R  A  T  I  O  N  S
R  E  I  E  E  D  E  M  A  U  R  O  R  Q
T  L  M  T  C  R  U  L  R  F  S  E  O  Y
C  C  U  S  Z  A  W  E  K  A  T  N  I  X
E  O  Z  O  T  T  A  N  A  U  N  M  F
L  F  K  D  P  I  O  I  W  W  Q  L  G  Q
E  N  I  L  C  O  O  H  O  W  S  B  X  S
N  J  X  A  L  N  F  S  U  N  L  J  J  J
O  C  U  V  S  A  L  G  T  I  S  C  Z  X
N  I  Z  L  L  D  Y  X  Q  Q  K  D  C  D
```

ADH	Edema	Nonelectrolytes
Aldosterone	Electrolytes	Output
Anions	Fluid balance	Overhydration
Cations	Homeostasis	Sodium
Dehydration	Intake	Thirst
Diuretic	Kidneys	Water

DID YOU KNOW?

The brain is a 3-pound greedy organ that demands 17% of all cardiac output and 20% of all available oxygen.

ACID/BASE BALANCE

Fill in the crossword puzzle.

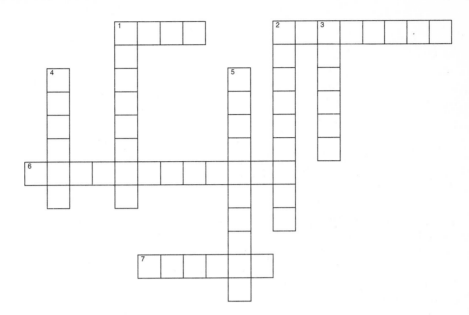

ACROSS

1. Substance with a pH lower than 7.0
2. Acid-base imbalance
6. Results from the excessive metabolism of fats in uncontrolled diabetics (two words)
7. Vomitus

DOWN

1. Substance with a pH higher than 7.0
2. Serious complication of vomiting
3. Emetic
4. Prevents a sharp change in the pH of fluids
5. Released as a waste product from working muscles (two words)

CHECK YOUR KNOWLEDGE

Multiple Choice

Circle the correct answer.

1. What happens as blood flows through lung capillaries?
   A. Carbonic acid in blood decreases.
   B. Hydrogen ions in blood decrease.
   C. Blood pH increases from venous to arterial blood.
   D. All of the above are true.

2. Which of the following organs is considered the most effective regulator of blood carbonic acid levels?
   A. Kidneys
   B. Intestines
   C. Lungs
   D. Stomach

3. Which of the following organs is considered the most effective regulator of blood pH?
   A. Kidneys
   B. Intestines
   C. Lungs
   D. Stomach

4. What is the pH of the blood?
   A. 7.00 to 8.00
   B. 6 25 to 7.45
   C. 7.65 to 7.85
   D. 7.35 to 7.45

5. If the ratio of sodium bicarbonate to carbonate ions is lowered (perhaps 10 to 1) and blood pH is also lowered, what is the condition called?
   A. Uncompensated metabolic acidosis
   B. Uncompensated metabolic alkalosis
   C. Compensated metabolic acidosis
   D. Compensated metabolic alkalosis

6. If a person hyperventilates for a given time period, which of the following will probably develop?
   A. Metabolic acidosis
   B. Metabolic alkalosis
   C. Respiratory acidosis
   D. Respiratory alkalosis

7. What happens when lactic acid dissociates in the blood?
   A. H+ is added to blood.
   B. pH is lowered.
   C. Acidosis results.
   D. All of the above happen.

8. Which of the following is true of metabolic alkalosis?
   A. It occurs in the case of prolonged vomiting.
   B. It results when the bicarbonate ion is present in excess.
   C. Therapy includes intravenous administration of normal saline.
   D. All of the above are true.

9. Which of the following is a characteristic of a buffer system in the body?
   A. It prevents drastic changes from occurring in body pH.
   B. It picks up both hydrogen and hydroxide ions.
   C. It is exemplified by the bicarbonate-carbonic acid system.
   D. All of the above are true.

10. In the presence of a strong acid, which of the following is true?
    A. Sodium bicarbonate will react to produce carbonic acid.
    B. Sodium bicarbonate will react to produce more sodium bicarbonate.
    C. Carbonic acid will react to produce sodium bicarbonate.
    D. Carbonic acid will react to form more carbonic acid.

Matching

Select the most correct answer from column B for each item in column A. (Only one answer is correct.)

Column A
_____ 11. pH lower than 7.0
_____ 12. pH higher than 7.0
_____ 13. Buffers
_____ 14. Decrease in respirations
_____ 15. Increase in respirations
_____ 16. Metabolic acidosis
_____ 17. Metabolic alkalosis
_____ 18. Lactic acid

_____ 19. Kidneys
_____ 20. Uncompensated metabolic acidosis

Column B
A. Bicarbonate deficit
B. Bicarbonate excess
C. Alkaline solution
D. "Fixed" acid
E. Respiratory acidosis
F. Respiratory alkalosis
G. Acidic solution
H. Lower-than-normal ratio of sodium bicarbonate to carbonic acid
I. Prevent sharp pH changes
J. Most effective regulators of body pH

CHAPTER 22

The Reproductive Systems

The reproductive system consists of those organs that participate in perpetuating the species. It is a unique body system in that its organs differ between the two sexes, and yet the goal of creating a new being is the same. Of interest also is the fact that this system is the only one not necessary to the survival of the individual, and yet survival of the species depends on the proper functioning of the reproductive organs. The male reproductive system is divided into the external genitals, the testes, the duct system, and accessory glands. The testes, or gonads, are considered essential organs because they produce the sex cells, sperm, which join with the female sex cells, ova, to form a new human being. They also secrete the male sex hormone, testosterone, which is responsible for the physical transformation of a boy to a man.

Sperm are formed in the testes by the seminiferous tubules. From there they enter a long narrow duct, the epididymis. They continue onward through the vas deferens into the ejaculatory duct, down the urethra, and out of the body. Throughout this journey, various glands secrete substances that add motility to the sperm and create a chemical environment conducive to reproduction.

The female reproductive system is truly extraordinary and diverse. It produces ova, receives the penis and sperm during intercourse, is the site of conception, houses and nourishes the embryo during prenatal development, and nourishes the infant after birth.

Because of its diversity, the physiology of the female is generally considered to be more complex than that of the male. Much of the activity of this system revolves around the menstrual cycle and the monthly preparation that the female undergoes for a possible pregnancy.

The organs of this system are divided into essential organs and accessory organs of reproduction. The essential organs of the female are the ovaries. Just as with the male, the essential organs of the female are referred to as the *gonads*. The gonads of both sexes produce the sex cells. In the male, the gonads produce the sperm and in the female they produce the ova. The gonads are also responsible for producing the hormones in each sex necessary for the appearance of the secondary sex characteristics.

The menstrual cycle of the female typically covers a period of 28 days. Each cycle consists of three phases: the menstrual period, the postmenstrual phase, and the premenstrual phase. Changes in the blood levels of the hormones that are responsible for the menstrual cycle also cause physical and emotional changes in the female. Knowledge of these phenomena and this system, in both the male and the female, are necessary to complete your understanding of the reproductive system.

TOPICS FOR REVIEW

Before progressing to Chapter 23 you should familiarize yourself with the structure and function of the organs of the male and female reproductive systems. Your review should include emphasis on the gross and microscopic structure of the testes and the production of sperm and testosterone. Your study should continue by tracing the pathway of a sperm cell from formation to expulsion from the body.

You should then familiarize yourself with the structure and function of the organs of the female reproductive system. Your review should include emphasis on the development of mature ova from ovarian follicles, and should additionally concentrate on the phases and occurrences in a typical 28-day menstrual cycle. Finally, a review of the common disorders occurring in both male and female reproductive systems is necessary to complete the study of this chapter.

MALE REPRODUCTIVE SYSTEM
STRUCTURAL PLAN

Match the term on the left with the proper selection on the right.

Group A

_____ 1.	Testes	A.	Fertilized ovum
_____ 2.	Spermatozoa	B.	Accessory organ
_____ 3.	Ova	C.	Male sex cell
_____ 4.	Penis	D.	Gonads
_____ 5.	Zygote	E.	Gamete

Group B

_____ 6.	Testes	A.	Cowper's gland
_____ 7.	Bulbourethral	B.	Scrotum
_____ 8.	Asexual	C.	Essential organ
_____ 9.	External genital	D.	Single parent
_____ 10.	Prostate	E.	Accessory organ

 If you have had difficulty with this section, review pages 653-655.

TESTES

Circle the correct answer.

11. The testes are surrounded by a tough membrane called the:
    A. Ductus deferens
    B. Tunica albuginea
    C. Septum
    D. Seminiferous membrane

12. The _____ lie near the septa that separate the lobules.
    A. Ductus deferens
    B. Sperm
    C. Interstitial cells
    D. Nerves

13. Sperm are found in the walls of the _____.
    A. Seminiferous tubule
    B. Interstitial cells
    C. Septum
    D. Blood vessels

14. The scrotum provides an environment that is approximately _____ for the testes.
    A. The same as the body temperature
    B. 5 degrees warmer than the body temperature
    C. 3 degrees warmer than the body temperature
    D. 3 degrees cooler than the body temperature

15. The _____ produce(s) testosterone.
    A. Seminiferous tubules
    B. Prostate gland
    C. Bulbourethral gland
    D. Pituitary gland
    E. Interstitial cells

16. The part of the sperm that contains genetic information that will be inherited is the:
    A. Tail
    B. Neck
    C. Middle piece
    D. Head
    E. Acrosome

17. Which one of the following is *not* a function of testosterone?
    A. It causes a deepening of the voice.
    B. It promotes the development of the male accessory organs.
    C. It has a stimulatory effect on protein catabolism.
    D. It causes greater muscular development and strength.

18. Sperm production is called:
    A. Spermatogonia
    B. Spermatids
    C. Spermatogenesis
    D. Spermatocyte

19. The section of the sperm that contains enzymes that enable it to break down the covering of the ovum and permit entry should contact occur is the:
    A. Acrosome
    B. Midpiece
    C. Tail
    D. Stem

Fill in the blanks.

The (20) _____ are the gonads of the male. From puberty on, the seminiferous tubules are continuously forming (21) _____. Any of these cells may join with the female sex cell, the (22) _____ to become a new human being. Another function of the testes is to secrete the male hormone (23) _____, that transforms a boy to a man. This hormone is secreted by the (24) _____ _____ of the testes. A good way to remember testosterone's functions is to think of it as "the (25) _____ hormone" and "the (26) _____ hormone."

▷ *If you have had difficulty with this section, review pages 655-659.*

REPRODUCTIVE DUCTS
ACCESSORY OR SUPPORTIVE SEX GLANDS
EXTERNAL GENITALS

Choose the correct term and write its letter in the space next to the appropriate definition below.

_____ 27.	Continuation of ducts that start in the epididymis	A. Epididymis
_____ 28.	Erectile tissue	B. Ductus (vas) deferens
_____ 29.	Also known as *bulbourethral*	C. Ejaculatory duct
_____ 30.	Narrow tube that lies along the top and behind the testes	D. Prepuce
_____ 31.	Doughnut-shaped gland beneath the bladder	E. Seminal vesicles
_____ 32.	Point where ductus (vas) deferens joins the duct from the seminal vesicle	F. Prostate gland
_____ 33.	Mixture of sperm and secretions of accessory sex glands	G. Cowper's gland
_____ 34.	Contributes 60% of the seminal fluid volume	H. Corpus spongiosum
_____ 35.	Removed during circumcision	I. Semen
_____ 36.	External genitalia	J. Scrotum

▷ *If you have had difficulty with this section, review pages 659-662.*

DISORDERS OF THE MALE REPRODUCTIVE SYSTEM

Fill in the blanks.

37. Decreased sperm production is called _____.

38. Testes normally descend into the scrotum about _____
    _____ before birth.

39. If a baby is born with undescended testes, a condition called _____ re-
    sults.

40. A common noncancerous condition of the prostate in older men is known as
    _____ _____
    _____.

41. _____ is a condition in which the foreskin fits so tightly over the glans
    that it cannot retract.

42. Failure to achieve an erection of the penis is called _____.

43. An accumulation of fluid in the scrotum is known as a _____.

44. An _____ _____ results when the
    intestines push through the weak area of the abdominal wall, which separates the abdominopelvic cavity
    from the scrotum.

45. The PSA test is a screening test for cancer of the _____.

▷ *If you have had difficulty with this section, review pages 662-665.*

FEMALE REPRODUCTIVE SYSTEM
STRUCTURAL PLAN

Match the term on the left with the proper selection on the right.

_____ 46. Ovaries   A. Genitals
_____ 47. Vagina   B. Accessory sex gland
_____ 48. Bartholin's   C. Accessory duct
_____ 49. Vulva   D. Gonads
_____ 50. Ova   E. Sex cell

Write the letter of the correct description in the blank next to the appropriate structure.

A. External structure   B. Internal structure

_____ 51. Mons pubis
_____ 52. Vagina
_____ 53. Labia majora
_____ 54. Uterine tubes
_____ 55. Vestibule
_____ 56. Clitoris
_____ 57. Labia minora
_____ 58. Ovaries

▷ *If you have had difficulty with this section, review pages 664-671.*

OVARIES

Fill in the blanks.

The ovaries are the (59) _____ of the female. They have two main functions. The first is the production of the female sex cell. This process is called (60) _____. The specialized type of cell division that occurs during sexual cell reproduction is known as (61) _____. The ovum is the body's largest cell and has (62) _____ the number of chromosomes found in other body cells. At the time of (63) _____, the sex cells from both parents fuse and (64) _____ chromosomes are united. The second major function of the ovaries is to secrete the sex hormones (65) _____ and (66) _____. Estrogen is the sex hormone that causes the development and maintenance of the female (67) _____ _____ _____. Progesterone acts with estrogen to help initiate the (68) _____ _____ in girls entering (69) _____.

▷ *If you have had difficulty with this section, review pages 665-668.*

FEMALE REPRODUCTIVE DUCTS

Write the letter of the correct structure in the blank next to the appropriate definition.

A. Uterine tubes   B. Uterus   C. Vagina

_____ 70. Most ectopic pregnancies

_____ 71. Lining known as *endometrium*

_____ 72. Terminal end of birth canal

_____ 73. Site of menstruation

_____ 74. Fringelike projections called *fimbriae*

_____ 75. Consists of body, fundus, and cervix

_____ 76. Site of fertilization

_____ 77. Also known as *oviduct*

_____ 78. Entrance way for sperm

▷ *If you have had difficulty with this section, review pages 668-670.*

ACCESSORY OR SUPPORTIVE SEX GLANDS
EXTERNAL GENITALS

Match the term on the left with the proper selection on the right.

Group A

_____ 79. Bartholin's gland   A. Colored area around the nipple

_____ 80. Breasts   B. Grapelike clusters of milk-secreting cells

_____ 81. Alveoli   C. Drain alveoli

_____ 82. Lactiferous ducts   D. Secretes lubricating fluid

_____ 83. Areola   E. Primarily fat tissue

Group B

_____ 84. Mons pubis   A. "Large lips"

_____ 85. Labia majora   B. Area between the vaginal opening and the anus

_____ 86. Clitoris   C. Surgical procedure

_____ 87. Perineum   D. Composed of erectile tissue

_____ 88. Episiotomy   E. Pad of fat over the symphysis pubis

▶ *If you have had difficulty with this section, review pages 670-672.*

MENSTRUAL CYCLE

If the statement is true, write "T" in the answer blank. If the statement is false, correct the statement by circling the incorrect term and inserting the correct term in the answer blank.

_____ 89. *Climacteric* is the scientific name for the beginning of the menses.

_____ 90. As a general rule, several ovum mature each month during the 30 to 40 years that a woman has menstrual periods.

_____ 91. Ovulation occurs 28 days before the next menstrual period begins.

_____ 92. The first day of ovulation is considered the first day of the cycle.

_____ 93. A woman's fertile period lasts only a few days out of each month.

_____ 94. The control of the menstrual cycle lies in the posterior pituitary gland.

Write the letter of the correct hormone in the blank next to the appropriate description.

A. FSH   B. LH

_____ 95. Ovulating hormone

_____ 96. Secreted during first days of menstrual cycle

_____ 97. Secreted after estrogen level of blood increases

_____ 98. Causes final maturation of follicle and ovum

_____ 99. Birth control pills suppress this one

▶ *If you have had difficulty with this section, review pages 672-675.*

DISORDERS OF THE FEMALE REPRODUCTIVE SYSTEM

Choose the correct response.

_____ 100. Often occurs from STDs or from a "yeast infection"

_____ 101. Benign tumor of smooth muscle and fibrous connective tissue. Also known as a *fibroid tumor*

_____ 102. Yeast infection characterized by leukorrhea

_____ 103. Inflammation of an ovary

_____ 104. Benign lumps in one or both breasts

_____ 105. Venereal diseases

_____ 106. Results from pathogenic organisms transmitted from another person; e.g., STD

_____ 107. Painful menstruation

_____ 108. Asymptomatic in most women and nearly all men

_____ 109. Results from a hormonal imbalance rather than from an infection or disease condition

_____ 110. Screening test for cervical cancer

_____ 111. Causes blisters on the skin of the genitals; the blisters may disappear temporarily, but recur, especially as a result of stress

A. Candidiasis
B. Dysmenorrhea

C. Exogenous infections
D. DUB
E. Myoma
F. Vaginitis
G. Sexually transmitted diseases (STDs)
H. Oophoritis
I. Fibrocystic disease
J. Pap smear

K. Genital herpes
L. Trichomoniasis

▷ *If you have had difficulty with this section, review pages 675-682.*

APPLYING WHAT YOU KNOW

112. Mr. Belinki is going into the hospital for the surgical removal of his testes. As a result of this surgery, will Mr. Belinki be impotent?

113. When baby Christopher was born, the pediatrician, Dr. Self, discovered that his left testicle had not descended into the scrotum. If this situation is not corrected soon, might baby Christopher be sterile or impotent?

114. Wilma contracted gonorrhea. By the time she made an appointment to see her doctor, it had spread to her abdominal organs. How is this possible when gonorrhea is a disease of the reproductive system?

115. Dr. Sullivan advised Mrs. Harlan to have a bilateral oophorectomy. Is this a sterilization procedure? Will she experience menopause?

116. Mrs. Kelly had a total hysterectomy. Will she experience menopause?

117. Word Find

Can you find the 18 terms from this chapter that are listed below? Words may be spelled top to bottom, bottom to top, right to left, left to right, or diagonally.

```
M  K  O  V  I  D  U  C  T  S  E  D  H  G
S  E  I  R  A  V  O  I  F  U  T  G  L  L
I  N  H  Z  H  M  P  M  K  O  H  I  C  W
D  D  V  A  S  D  E  F  E  R  E  N  S  H
I  O  A  C  C  I  P  J  V  E  H  Y  D  S
H  M  G  R  R  B  M  N  X  F  G  Y  I  O
C  E  I  O  O  E  Z  Y  T  I  C  S  T  E
R  T  N  S  T  P  S  D  D  N  O  V  A  D
O  R  A  O  U  W  E  B  A  I  J  S  M  Z
T  I  C  M  M  E  Y  N  E  M  D  L  R  V
P  U  A  E  U  D  G  M  I  E  H  I  E  H
Y  M  O  T  C  E  T  A  T  S  O  R  P  B
R  P  E  E  R  M  N  E  G  O  R  T  S  E
C  O  W  P  E  R  S  I  N  X  K  E  A  P
```

Acrosome	Meiosis	Scrotum
Cowpers	Ovaries	Seminiferous
Cryptorchidism	Oviducts	Sperm
Endometrium	Penis	Spermatids
Epididymis	Pregnancy	Vagina
Estrogen	Prostatectomy	Vas deferens

DID YOU KNOW?

The testes produce approximately 50 million sperm per day. Every 2 to 3, months they produce enough cells to populate the entire earth.

There are an estimated 925,000 daily occurrences of STD transmission and 550,000 daily pregnancies worldwide.

The United States has one of the highest teen pregnancy rates of all industrialized nations. Rates in France, Germany, and Japan are four times lower.

REPRODUCTIVE SYSTEM

Fill in the crossword puzzle.

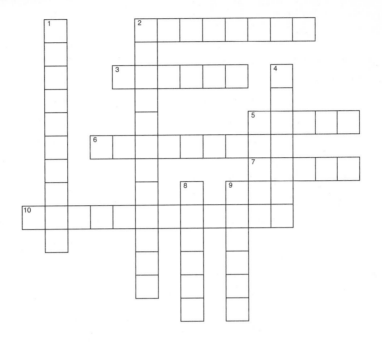

ACROSS

2. Female erectile tissue
3. Colored area around nipple
5. Male reproductive fluid
6. Sex cells
7. External genitalia
10. Male sex hormone

DOWN

1. Failure to have a menstrual period
2. Surgical removal of foreskin
4. Foreskin
8. Menstrual period
9. Essential organs of reproduction

CHECK YOUR KNOWLEDGE

Multiple Choice

Circle the correct answer.

1. What is the membrane that may cover the vaginal opening of the female called?
   A. Hymen
   B. Mons pubis
   C. Labia
   D. Clitoris

2. Which of the following statements is/are true of the menstrual cycle?
   A. Estrogen levels are lowest at the time of ovulation.
   B. Progesterone levels are highest at the time of ovulation.
   C. FSH levels are highest during the proliferation phase.
   D. None of the above are true.

3. A fluid mixture called *semen* could contain which of the following?
    A. Sperm cells
    B. Secretion from the prostate
    C. Secretions from the seminal vesicles
    D. All of the above

4. What is the failure of the testes to descend into the scrotum before birth called?
    A. Cryptococcoses
    B. Coccidioidomycosis
    C. Cryptorchidism
    D. Cholelithiasis

5. Which of the following is *not* an accessory organ of the female reproductive system?
    A. Breast
    B. Bartholin's glands
    C. Ovary
    D. All of the above are accessory organs

6. Which of the following structures can be referred to as *male gonads*?
    A. Testes
    B. Epididymis
    C. Vas deferens
    D. All of the above

7. Sperm cells are suspended outside the body cavity so as to do which of the following?
    A. Protect them from trauma
    B. Keep them at a cooler temperature
    C. Keep them supplied with a greater number of blood vessels
    D. Protect them from infection

8. What is the removal of the foreskin from the glans penis called?
    A. Vasectomy
    B. Sterilization
    C. Circumcision
    D. Ligation

9. What is the colored area around the nipple of the breast called?
    A. Areola
    B. Lactiferous duct
    C. Alveoli
    D. None of the above

10. Which of the following is true in the postmenstrual phase of the menstrual cycle?
    A. The endometrium is being repaired.
    B. Luteinizing hormone is secreted.
    C. Progesterone is being secreted.
    D. All of the above are true.

Completion

Complete the following statements using the terms listed below.

A. Clitoris
B. Endometrium
C. Ectopic
D. Corpus luteum

E. Menses
F. Epididymis
G. Hysterectomy
H. Prostate

I. FSH (follicle-stimulating hormone)
J. Ovulation
K. Scrotum
L. Testosterone

11. A pregnancy resulting from the implantation of a fertilized ovum in any location other than the uterus is called _____.

12. Interstitial cells of the testes function to produce _____.

13. The doughnut-shaped accessory organ or gland that surrounds the male urethra is called the _____.

14. Surgical removal of the uterus is called _____.

15. The _____ houses sperm cells as they mature and develop their ability to swim.

16. The skin-covered, external pouch that contains the testes is called the _____.

17. The lining of the uterus is called _____.

18. The hormone progesterone is secreted by a structure called the _____.

19. Fertilization of an egg by a sperm can only occur around the time of _____.

20. From about the first to the seventh day of the menstrual cycle, the anterior pituitary gland secretes _____.

MALE REPRODUCTIVE ORGANS

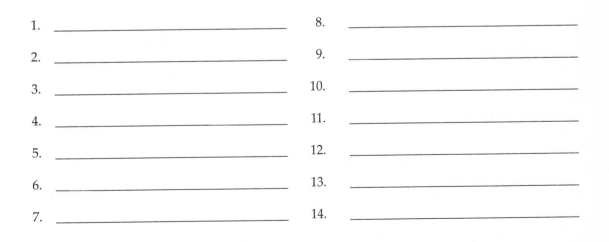

1. _____   8. _____

2. _____   9. _____

3. _____   10. _____

4. _____   11. _____

5. _____   12. _____

6. _____   13. _____

7. _____   14. _____

TUBULES OF TESTIS AND EPIDIDYMIS

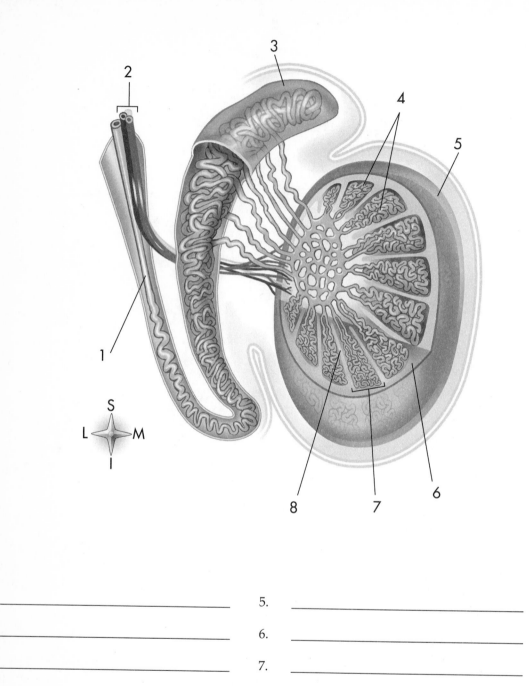

1. _____   5. _____

2. _____   6. _____

3. _____   7. _____

4. _____   8. _____

VULVA

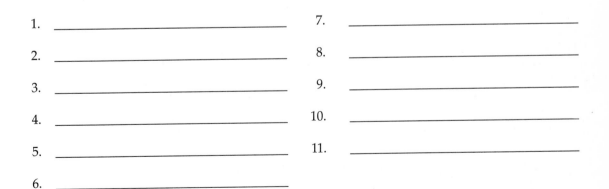

1. _____   7. _____

2. _____   8. _____

3. _____   9. _____

4. _____   10. _____

5. _____   11. _____

6. _____

BREAST

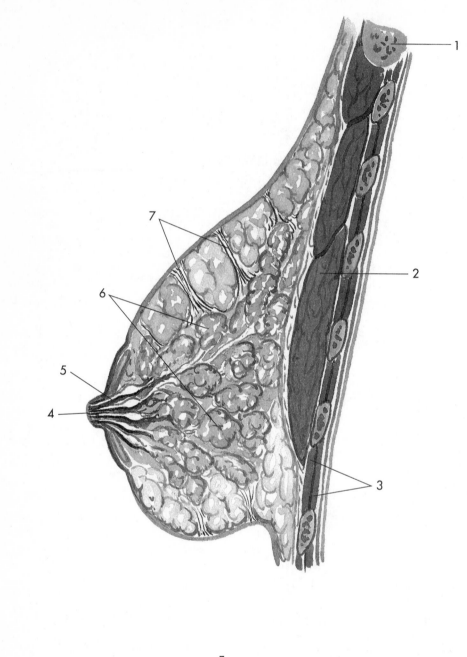

1. _____   5. _____

2. _____   6. _____

3. _____   7. _____

4. _____

FEMALE PELVIS

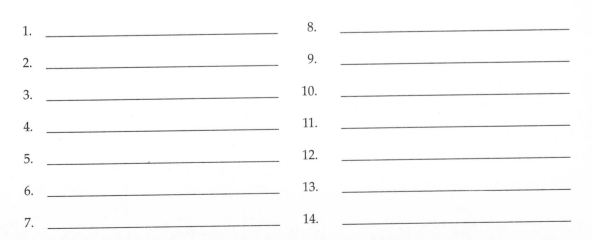

1. _____   8. _____

2. _____   9. _____

3. _____   10. _____

4. _____   11. _____

5. _____   12. _____

6. _____   13. _____

7. _____   14. _____

UTERUS AND ADJACENT STRUCTURES

1. _____

2. _____

3. _____

4. _____

5. _____

6. _____

7. _____

8. _____

9. _____

10. _____

11. _____

CHAPTER 23

Growth and Development

Millions of fragile microscopic sperm swim against numerous obstacles to reach the ova and create a new life. At birth, the newborn will fill his lungs with air and cry lustily, signaling to the world that he is ready to begin the cycle of life. This cycle will be marked by ongoing changes, periodic physical growth, and continuous development.

This chapter reviews the more significant events that occur in the normal growth and development of an individual from conception to death. Realizing that each person is unique, we nonetheless can discover amid all the complexities of humanity some constants that are understandable and predictable.

Knowledge of human growth and development is essential in understanding the commonalties that influence individuals as they pass through the cycle of life.

TOPICS FOR REVIEW

Before progressing to Chapter 24 you should have an understanding of the concept of development as a biological process. You should familiarize yourself with the major developmental changes from conception through older adulthood. The disorders of pregnancy should be emphasized as you review the chapter. Finally, your study should conclude with a review of the effects of aging on the body systems.

PRENATAL PERIOD
BIRTH OR PARTURITION

Fill in the blanks.

The prenatal stage of development begins at the time of (1) _____ and continues until (2) _____. The science of the development of an individual before birth is called (3) _____. Fertilization takes place in the outer third of the (4) _____. The fertilized ovum or (5) _____ begins to divide and in approximately 3 days forms a solid mass called a (6) _____. By the time it enters the uterus, it is a hollow ball of cells called a (7) _____. As it continues to develop, it forms a structure with two cavities. The (8) _____ _____ will become a fluid-filled sac for the embryo. The (9) _____ will develop into an important fetal membrane in the (10) _____.

Choose the correct term and write its letter in the space next to the appropriate definition below.

_____ 11. "Within a glass"

_____ 12. Inside germ layer

_____ 13. Before birth

_____ 14. Length of pregnancy

_____ 15. Fiberoptic viewing instrument

_____ 16. Process of birth

_____ 17. Surgical procedure in which a newborn is delivered through an incision in the abdomen and uterine wall

_____ 18. Study of how the primary germ layers develop into many different kinds of tissues

_____ 19. Fertilization until the end of the eighth week of gestation

_____ 20. Monitors progress of developing fetus

A. Laparoscope

B. Gestation

C. Antenatal

D. Histogenesis

E. C-section

F. Endoderm

G. In vitro

H. Parturition

I. Embryonic phase

J. Ultrasonogram

▷ *If you have had difficulty with this section, review pages 691-703 and page 705.*

DISORDERS OF PREGNANCY

If the statement is true, write "T" in the answer blank. If the statement is false, correct the statement by circling the incorrect term and inserting the correct term in the answer blank.

_____ 21. Many offspring are lost before implantation occurs, often for unknown reasons.

_____ 22. The most common type of ectopic pregnancy is a tubal pregnancy.

_____ 23. If the placenta grows too closely to the cervical opening a condition called *abruptio placentae* results.

_____ 24. Separation of the placenta from the uterine wall in a pregnancy of 20 weeks or more is known as *placenta previa*.

_____ 25. Toxemia of pregnancy is also known as *puerperal fever*.

_____ 26. After 20 weeks, delivery of a lifeless infant is termed a *miscarriage*.

_____ 27. Acquired birth defects result from agents called *teratogens* that disrupt normal histogenesis and organogenesis.

▷ *If you have had difficulty with this section, review pages 703-706.*

POSTNATAL PERIOD

Circle the correct answer.

28. During the postnatal period:
   A. The head becomes proportionately smaller
   B. Thoracic and abdominal contours change from round to elliptical
   C. The legs become proportionately longer
   D. The trunk becomes proportionately shorter
   E. All of the above take place during the postnatal period

29. The period of infancy starts at birth and lasts about:
   A. 4 weeks
   B. 4 months
   C. 10 weeks
   D. 12 months
   E. 18 months

30. The lumbar curvature of the spine appears _____ months after birth.
    A. 1 to 10
    B. 5 to 8
    C. 8 to 12
    D. 11 to 15
    E. 12 to 18

31. During the first 4 months, the birth weight will:
    A. Double
    B. Triple
    C. Quadruple
    D. None of the above

32. At the end of the first year, the weight of the baby will have:
    A. Doubled
    B. Tripled
    C. Quadrupled
    D. None of the above

33. The infant is capable of following a moving object with its eyes at:
    A. 2 days
    B. 2 weeks
    C. 2 months
    D. 4 months
    E. 10 months

34. The infant can lift its head and raise its chest at:
    A. 2 months
    B. 3 months
    C. 4 months
    D. 10 months

35. The infant can crawl at:
    A. 2 months
    B. 3 months
    C. 4 months
    D. 10 months
    E. 12 months

36. The infant can stand alone at:
    A. 2 months
    B. 3 months
    C. 4 months
    D. 10 months
    E. 12 months

37. The permanent teeth, with the exception of the third molar, have all erupted by age _____ years.
    A. 6
    B. 8
    C. 12
    D. 14
    E. None of the above

38. Puberty starts at age _____ years in boys.
    A. 10 to 13
    B. 12 to 14
    C. 14 to 16
    D. None of the above

39. Most girls begin breast development at about age:
    A. 8
    B. 9
    C. 10
    D. 11
    E. 12

40. The growth spurt is generally complete by age _____ in males.
    A. 14
    B. 15
    C. 16
    D. 18

41. An average age at which girls begin to menstruate is _____ years.
    A. 10 to 12
    B. 11 to 12
    C. 12 to 13
    D. 13 to 14
    E. 14 to 15

42. The first sign of puberty in boys is:
    A. Facial hair
    B. Increased muscle mass
    C. Pubic hair
    D. Deepening of the voice
    E. Enlargement of the testicles

Write the letter of the correct word in the blank next to the appropriate definition.

_____ 43. Begins at birth and lasts until death

_____ 44. Concerned with the diagnosis and treatment of disorders of the newborn

_____ 45. Teenage years

_____ 46. From the end of infancy to puberty

_____ 47. Baby teeth

_____ 48. First 4 weeks of infancy

_____ 49. Secondary sexual characteristics occur

_____ 50. Study of aging

_____ 51. Older adulthood

A. Neonatology
B. Neonatal
C. Adolescence
D. Deciduous
E. Puberty
F. Postnatal
G. Gerontology
H. Childhood
I. Senescence

▶ *If you have had difficulty with this section, review pages 706-710.*

EFFECTS OF AGING

Fill in the blanks.

52. Old bones develop indistinct and shaggy margins with spurs; a process called
_____.

53. A degenerative joint disease common in the aged is _____.

54. The number of _____ units in the kidney decreases by almost 50% between the ages of 30 and 75.

55. In old age, respiratory efficiency decreases and a condition known as
_____ _____ results.

56. Fatty deposits accumulate in blood vessels as we age, and the result is
_____, which narrows the passageway for the flow of blood.

57. Hardening of the arteries, or _____, occurs during the aging process.

58. Another term for high blood pressure is _____.

59. Hardening of the lens is _____.

60. If the lens becomes cloudy and impairs vision, it is called a _____.

61. _____ causes an increase in the pressure within the eyeball and may result in blindness.

▶ *If you have had difficulty with this section, review pages 710-714.*

UNSCRAMBLE THE WORDS

62. **A N N F C Y I**

    ⬭ ⬭ ▢ ▢ ▢ ▢

63. **N A A L T T S O P**

    ▢ ▢ ▢ ▢ ⬭ ▢ ⬭ ▢ ⬭

64. **O G S S N E G R A O N E I**

    ▢ ⬭ ▢ ⬭ ▢ ▢ ▢ ⬭ ▢ ▢ ▢ ⬭

65. **G T E Y Z O**

    ⬭ ▢ ▢ ⬭ ▢

66. **H D O O L H C I D**

    ▢ ⬭ ▢ ▢ ▢ ⬭ ▢

Take the circled letters, unscramble them, and fill in the statement.

The secret to Farmer Brown's prize pumpkin crop.

67. ▢ ▢ ▢ ▢ ▢ ▢ ▢ ▢ ▢ ▢ ▢ ▢ ▢

The secret is in the bag

APPLYING WHAT YOU KNOW

68. Billy's mother told the pediatrician during his 1-year visit that Billy had tripled his birth weight, was crawling actively, and could stand alone. Is Billy's development normal, retarded, or advanced?

69. John is 70 years old. He has always enjoyed food and has had a hearty appetite. Lately, however, he has complained that food "just doesn't taste as good anymore." What might be a possible explanation?

70. Mr. Gaylor has noticed hearing problems but only under certain circumstances. He has difficulty with certain tones, especially high or low tones, but has no problem with everyday conversation. What might be a possible explanation?

71. Mrs. Lowell gave birth to twin girls. The obstetrician, Dr. Sullivan, advised Mr. Lowell that even though the girls looked identical, they were really fraternal twins. How was he able to deduce this?

72. Word Find

Can you find the 13 terms from this chapter that are listed below? Words may be spelled top to bottom, bottom to top, right to left, left to right, or diagonally.

```
F C M P O D N P P A G M J N Z
K E C N E C S E L O D A G G M
I N R B U X T K D A Y Q T F R
L D L T O M S D W A E Z B F E
Z O B A I S P M A L C E E R P
W D I M P L A N T A T I O N L
H E N M K A I T E P D K S X A
W R G A S A R Z R N T Q P Y C
L M Q S I J O O A U B F G T E
R T N T B N G E S T A T I O N
L A T I N E G N O C I T F Z T
D C B T R L A S G C O O R R A
E N O I T I R U T R A P N S B
N V A S N N E G O T A R E T E
```

Adolescence	Implantation	Placenta
Congenital	Laparoscope	Preeclampsia
Endoderm	Mastitis	Progeria
Fertilization	Parturition	Teratogen
Gestation		

DID YOU KNOW?

Brain cells do not regenerate. One beer permanently destroys 10,000 cells.

GROWTH/DEVELOPMENT

Fill in the crossword puzzle.

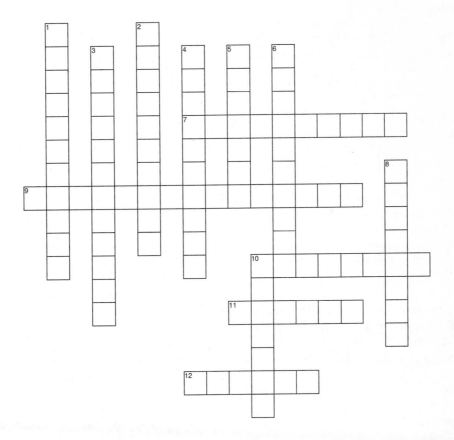

ACROSS	DOWN

ACROSS

7. Old age
9. Fatty deposit buildup on walls of arteries
10. Cloudy lens
11. Name of zygote after 3 days
12. Fertilized ovum

DOWN

1. Process of birth
2. Science of the development of the individual before birth
3. Study of how germ layers develop into tissues
4. Name of zygote after implantation
5. First 4 weeks of infancy
6. Hardening of the lens
8. Eye disease marked by increased pressure in the eyeball
10. Will develop into a fetal membrane in the placenta

CHECK YOUR KNOWLEDGE

Multiple Choice

Circle the correct answer.

1. When the human embryo is a hollow ball of cells consisting of an outer cell layer and an inner cell mass, what is it called?
   A. Morula
   B. Chorion
   C. Blastocyst
   D. Zygote

2. Degenerative changes in the urinary system that accompany old age include which of the following?
   A. Decreased capacity of the bladder and the inability to empty or void completely
   B. Decrease in the number of nephrons
   C. Less blood flow through the kidneys
   D. All of the above

3. The frontal and maxillary sinuses of the facial region acquire permanent placement or develop fully when the individual is in a stage of development known as which of the following?
   A. Infancy
   B. Childhood
   C. Adolescence
   D. Adulthood

4. The first 4 weeks of human life following birth are referred to as which of the following?
   A. Neonatal
   B. Infancy
   C. Prenatal
   D. Embryonic

5. Any hardening of the arteries is referred to as which of the following?
   A. Angioma
   B. Atherosclerosis
   C. Angina
   D. Arteriosclerosis

6. Which of the following is characteristic of the disorder called *presbyopia*?
   A. It is very characteristic of old age.
   B. It causes farsightedness in some individuals.
   C. It is characterized by the lens in the eye becoming hard and losing its elasticity.
   D. All of the above are true.

7. The three most important "low tech" methods for improving the quality of life as you age are:
   A. Healthy diet, exercise, and stress management
   B. A healthy diet, marriage, and money
   C. A healthy diet, good job, and living in the suburbs
   D. A healthy diet, weight management, and exercise

8. Which of the following events, if any, is *not* characteristic of adolescence?
   A. Bone closure occurs.
   B. Secondary sexual characteristics develop.
   C. Very rapid growth occurs.
   D. All of the above events are characteristic of adolescence.

9. Which of the following events is *not* characteristic of the prenatal period of development?
   A. Blastocyst is formed.
   B. Histogenesis occurs.
   C. Bone closure occurs.
   D. Amniotic cavity is formed.

10. Which of the following structures is derived from ectoderm?
    A. The lining of the lungs
    B. The brain
    C. The kidneys
    D. All of the above

Matching

Select the correct answer from column B for each item in column A. (Only one answer is correct.)

Column A

_____ 11. Arteriosclerosis

_____ 12. Atherosclerosis

_____ 13. Parturition

_____ 14. Cataract

_____ 15. Adolescence

_____ 16. Amniotic sac

_____ 17. Glaucoma

_____ 18. Senescence

_____ 19. Hypertension

_____ 20. Placenta

Column B

A. High blood pressure

B. Chorion

C. Birth

D. "Bag of waters"

E. Hardening of arteries

F. Degeneration

G. Fat accumulation in arteries

H. Secondary sexual characteristics

I. Clouding of eye lens

J. High eye pressure

FERTILIZATION AND IMPLANTATION

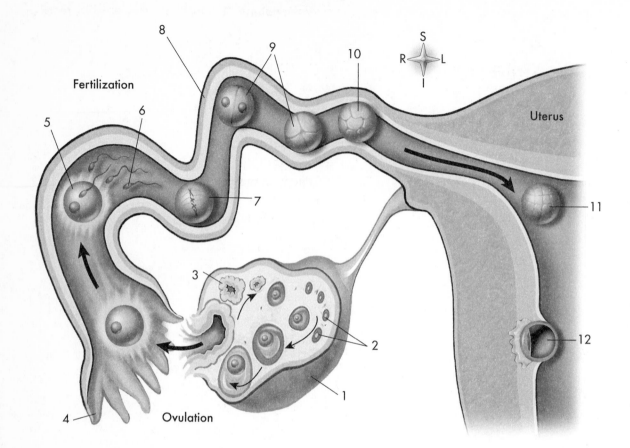

1. _____
2. _____
3. _____
4. _____
5. _____
6. _____

7. _____
8. _____
9. _____
10. _____
11. _____
12. _____

Genetics and Genetic Diseases

L ook around your classroom and you will notice various combinations of hair color, eye color, body size, skin tone, hair texture, sex, etc. Everyone has unique body features and this phenomenon alerts us to the marvel of genetics. Independent units, called *genes*, are responsible for the inheritance of biological traits. Genes determine the structure and function of the human body by producing specific regulatory enzymes. Some genes are dominant and some are recessive. Dominant genes produce traits that appear in the offspring and recessive genes have traits that do not appear in the offspring when they are masked by a dominant gene.

Gene therapy is one of the latest advances of science. This revolutionary branch of medicine combines current technology with genetic research to unlock the secrets of the human body. Daily discoveries into the prevention, diagnosis, treatment, and cure of diseases and disorders are being revealed as a result of genetic therapy. Knowledge of genetics is necessary to understand the basic mechanism by which traits are transmitted from parents to offspring.

TOPICS FOR REVIEW

Your review of this chapter should include an understanding of chromosomes, genes, and gene expression. You should continue your study with a knowledge of common genetic diseases. Finally, your review should conclude with an understanding of the prevention and treatment of genetic diseases.

GENETICS AND HUMAN DISEASE
CHROMOSOMES AND GENES
HUMAN GENOME

Match the term on the left with the proper selection on the right.

_____ 1.	Gene	A.	DNA molecule
_____ 2.	Chromosome	B.	Male or female reproductive cell
_____ 3.	Gamete	C.	Special form of nuclear division
_____ 4.	Meiosis	D.	Formed by union of sperm and ovum at conception
_____ 5.	Zygote	E.	Distinct code within a DNA molecule
_____ 6.	Genome	F.	Adenine
_____ 7.	Genomics	G.	Entire collection of genetic material in each typical cell
_____ 8.	Proteomics	H.	Cartoon of a chromosome
_____ 9.	Ideogram	I.	Analysis of the genome's code
_____ 10.	Nucleotide base	J.	Analysis of the proteins encoded by the genome

▷ *If you have had difficulty with this section, review pages 723-726.*

GENE EXPRESSION

Fill in the blanks.

After experimentation with pea plants, Mendel discovered that each inherited trait is controlled by two sets
of similar (11) _____, one from each parent. He also noted that some genes
are (12) _____ and some are (13) _____.
In the example of albinism, a person with the gene combination of Aa is said to be a genetic
(14) _____. If two different dominant genes occur together a form of dominance called (15) _____ exists. (16) _____
chromosomes do not have matching structures. If an individual has the sex chromosomes XX, that person will
have the sexual characteristics of a (17) _____.
(18) _____ simply means "change." A
(19) _____ _____ is a change in the genetic code.

▷ *If you have had difficulty with this section, review pages 726-732.*

GENETIC DISEASES

*Choose the term that applies to each of the following descriptions. Place the letter for the term in the
appropriate answer blank.*

_____ 20. Caused by recessive genes in chromosome pair 7	A.	Single-gene disease
_____ 21. Results in total blindness by age 30	B.	Nondisjunction
_____ 22. Disease conditions that result from the combined effects of inheritance and environmental factors	C.	Monosomy
_____ 23. Results from a failure to produce the enzyme phenylalanine hydroxylase	D.	Leber's hereditary optic neuropathy
_____ 24. Presence of only one autosome instead of a pair	E.	Cystic fibrosis
_____ 25. Usually caused by trisomy of chromosome 21	F.	Phenylketonuria
_____ 26. Cystic fibrosis is an example	G.	Down syndrome
_____ 27. Results from nondisjunction of chromosomes and typically has the XXY pattern	H.	Klinefelter's syndrome
_____ 28. Term used to describe what happens when a pair of chromosomes fails to separate	I.	Turner's syndrome
_____ 29. Sometimes called *XO syndrome*, it is treated with hormone therapy	J.	Genetic predisposition

▷ *If you have had difficulty with this section, review pages 732-736.*

PREVENTION AND TREATMENT OF GENETIC DISEASES

Circle the correct answer.

30. A pedigree is a chart that can be used to determine:
    A. Genetic relationships in a family over several generations
    B. The possibility of producing offspring with certain genetic disorders
    C. The possibility of a person developing a genetic disorder late in life
    D. All of the above
    E. None of the above

31. The Punnett Square is a grid used to determine:
    A. Genetic disorders
    B. The probability of inheriting genetic traits
    C. Proper gene replacement therapy
    D. The necessity for amniocentesis

32. Some forms of cancer are thought to be caused, at least in part, by abnormal genes called:
    A. Cancercytes
    B. Trisomy
    C. Oncogenes
    D. Autosomes

33. When producing a karyotype, the most common source of cells for the sample is the:
    A. Vagina
    B. Rectum
    C. Lining of the cheek
    D. Throat

34. An ultrasound transducer is used during amniocentesis to:
    A. Create a sharper image
    B. Take measurements during the procedure
    C. Prevent damaging rays during the procedure
    D. Guide the tip of the needle to prevent placental damage

35. Electrophoresis is a process that:
    A. Provides a method for DNA analysis
    B. Means electric separation
    C. Is the basis for DNA fingerprinting
    D. All of the above

36. The use of genetic therapy began in 1990 with a group of young children who had:
    A. AIDS
    B. Adenosine deaminase deficiency
    C. Hemophilia
    D. Cystic fibrosis

If the statement is true, write "T" in the answer blank. If the statement is false, correct the statement by circling the incorrect term and inserting the correct term in the answer blank.

_____ 37. Chorionic villus sampling is a procedure in which cells that surround a young embryo are collected through the opening of the cervix.

_____ 38. Karyotyping is the process used for DNA fingerprinting.

_____ 39. In amniocentesis, normal genes are introduced with the hope that they will add to the production of the needed protein.

_____ 40. Deficiency of adenosine deaminase results in severe combined immune deficiency.

_____ 41. One hypothesis that may explain some forms of cancer is known as the *tumor suppressor gene* hypothesis.

▶ *If you have had difficulty with this section, review pages 736-743.*

UNSCRAMBLE THE WORDS

42. **R C R R I E A**

43. **Y T S M O I R**

44. **E G N E**

45. **D P E R E G I E**

46. **S O E M C R O S H O M**

Take the circled letters, unscramble them, and fill in the statement.

How Bill made his fortune.

47.

APPLYING WHAT YOU KNOW

48. Steve's mother has a dominant gene for dark skin color. Steve's father has a dominant gene for light skin color. What color will Steve's skin most likely be?

49. Mr. and Mrs. Freund both carry recessive genes for cystic fibrosis. Using your knowledge of the Punnett square, estimate the probability of one of their offspring inheriting this condition.

50. Linda is pregnant and is over 40. She fears her age may predispose her baby to genetic disorders and she has sought the advice of a genetic counselor. What tests might the counselor suggest to alleviate Linda's fears?

51. Punnett Square

Fill in the Punnett square for the following genetic cases:

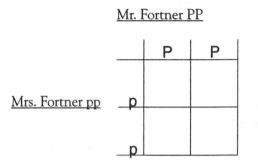

Mr. Fortner PP

Mrs. Fortner pp

Mr. Fortner has two dominant genes for brown eyes and Mrs. Fortner has two recessive genes for blue eyes.

a. The offspring of Mr. and Mrs. Fortner have a _____ % chance of having brown eyes and a _____ % chance of having blue eyes.

b. Will Mr. and Mrs. Fortner's offspring be carriers of blue eyes?

c. If Mr. and Mrs. Fortner's offspring mates with another offspring who is a carrier of blue eyes, what is the probability of the resulting offspring having blue eyes?

Draw your own Punnett Square to determine your answer.

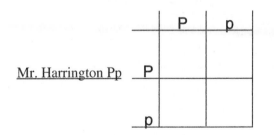

Mrs. Harrington Pp

Mr. Harrington Pp

Mr. and Mrs. Harrington are both carriers for albinism. Using the Punnett square, determine what percentage of Mr. and Mrs. Harrington's offspring will:

a. Have normal pigmentation _____

b. Be carriers _____

c. Have albinism _____

52.   Word Find

Can you find the 14 terms from this chapter that are listed below? Words may be spelled top to bottom, bottom to top, right to left, left to right, or diagonally.

```
N  J  A  T  E  T  O  G  Y  Z  S  F  I  H  Q
M  O  M  D  P  S  I  W  P  L  I  K  Y  E  K
S  M  N  P  E  E  F  Y  A  Z  S  A  X  M  C
F  A  I  D  V  M  M  Z  R  Z  O  R  P  O  L
H  R  O  J  I  O  E  U  E  I  I  Y  D  P  O
I  Q  C  M  S  S  O  L  H  Z  E  O  G  H  X
Y  J  E  O  S  O  J  Z  T  W  M  T  D  I  Q
G  E  N  I  E  M  C  U  E  I  E  Y  X  L  Q
A  O  T  G  C  O  P  K  N  E  J  P  I  I  G
M  P  E  M  E  R  D  A  E  C  P  E  J  A  I
E  D  S  I  R  H  N  C  G  B  T  Z  P  S  Y
T  G  I  D  U  C  G  C  P  X  H  I  F  G  X
E  W  S  R  E  I  R  R  A  C  V  I  O  H  S
S  W  V  B  K  R  C  R  Y  B  V  U  C  N  S
```

Amniocentesis	Gametes	Monosomy
Carrier	Gene therapy	Nondisjunction
Chromosomes	Hemophilia	Recessive
Codominance	Karyotype	Zygote
DNA	Meiosis	

DID YOU KNOW?

Scientists now believe the human body has 50,000 to 100,000 genes packed into just 46 chromosomes.

GENETICS

Fill in the crossword puzzle.

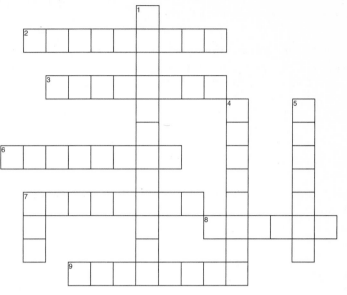

ACROSS

2. Name for the 22 pairs of matched chromosomes
3. Lack of melanin in the skin and eyes
6. Refers to genes that appear in the offspring
7. Chart that illustrates genetic relationships in a family over several generations
8. All genetic material in each cell
9. Scientific study of inheritance

DOWN

1. Trisomy 21 (two words)
4. Agents that cause genetic mutations
5. Triplet of autosomes rather than a pair
7. Excess of phenylketone in the urine (abbreviation)

CHECK YOUR KNOWLEDGE

Multiple Choice

Circle the correct answer.

1. Independent assortment of chromosomes ensures:
   A. Each offspring from a single set of parents is genetically unique
   B. At meiosis, each gamete receives the same number of chromosomes
   C. That the sex chromosomes always match
   D. An equal number of males and females are born

2. Which of the following statements is *not* true of a pedigree?
   A. They are useful to genetic counselors in predicting the possibility of producing offspring with genetic disorders.
   B. They may allow a person to determine his likelihood of developing a genetic disorder later in life.
   C. They indicate the occurrence of those family members affected by a trait, as well as carriers of the trait.
   D. All of the above are true of a pedigree.

3. The genes that cause albinism are:
   A. Codominant
   B. Dominant
   C. Recessive
   D. AA

4. During meiosis, matching pairs of chromosomes line up and exchange genes from their location to the same location on the other side; a process called:
   A. Gene linkage
   B. Crossing-over
   C. Cross-linkage
   D. Genetic variation

5. When a sperm cell unites with an ovum, a _____ is formed.
   A. Zygote
   B. Chromosome
   C. Gamete
   D. None of the above

6. DNA molecules can also be called:
   A. A chromatin strand
   B. A chromosome
   C. A and B
   D. None of the above

7. Sex-linked traits:
   A. Show up more often in females than in males
   B. Are nonsexual traits carried on sex chromosomes
   C. Are the result of genetic mutation
   D. All of the above

8. If a person has only X chromosomes, that person is:
   A. Missing essential proteins
   B. Abnormal
   C. Female
   D. Male

9. A karyotype:
   A. Can detect trisomy
   B. Is useful for diagnosing a tubal pregnancy
   C. Is frequently used as a tool in gene augmentation therapy
   D. Can detect the presence of oncogenes

10. Which of the following pairs is mismatched?
    A. SCID—gene therapy
    B. Turner's syndrome—trisomy
    C. PKU—recessive
    D. Cystic fibrosis—single-gene disease

Completion

Complete the following statements using the terms listed below.

A. Cystic fibrosis
B. Males
C. Phenylketonuria
D. Carrier
E. Genome
F. Females

G. Pedigree
H. Oncogenes
I. Karyotype
J. Tay-Sachs disease
K. Amniocentesis
L. Hemophilia

11. Abnormal genes called _____ are believed to be related to cancer.

12. Fetal tissue may be collected by a procedure called _____.

13. An abnormal accumulation of phenylalanine results in _____.

14. The entire collection of genetic material in each cell is called the _____.

15. _____ is caused by recessive genes in chromosome pair seven.

16. A _____ is a chart that illustrates genetic relationships over several generations.

17. A _____ is a person who has a recessive gene that is not expressed.

18. Absence of an essential lipid-producing enzyme may result in the recessive condition _____.

19. _____ is a recessive X-linked disorder.

20. Klinefelter's syndrome occurs in _____.

Answers to Exercises

CHAPTER 1
AN INTRODUCTION TO THE STRUCTURE AND FUNCTION OF THE BODY

Matching

1. D, p. 2
2. E, p. 2
3. A, p. 4
4. C, p. 4
5. B, p. 4

Matching

6. C, p. 4
7. A, p. 4
8. E, p. 4
9. D, p. 4
10. B, p. 4

Crossword

11. Superior
12. Inferior
13. Transverse
14. Ventral
15. Lateral
16. Medial
17. Distal

Did you notice that the answers were arranged as they appear on the human body?

Circle the Correct Answer

18. Inferior, p. 5
19. Anterior, p. 5
20. Lateral, p. 6
21. Proximal, p. 6
22. Superficial, p. 6
23. Equal, p. 6
24. Anterior and posterior, p. 6
25. Upper and lower, p. 6
26. Frontal, p. 6

Select the Correct Term

27. A, p. 6
28. B, p. 8
29. A, p. 6
30. A, p. 6
31. A, p. 6
32. B, p. 8
33. A, p. 6

Circle the One that Does Not Belong

34. Extremities (all others are part of the axial portions)
35. Cephalic (all others are part of the arm)
36. Plantar (all others are part of the face)
37. Carpal (all others are part of the leg or foot)
38. Tarsal (all others are part of the skull)

True or False

39. T
40. F (three stages), p. 7
41. T
42. F (they are not usually dissected), p. 7
43. F (during stage 3), p. 7
44. T

Fill in the Blanks

45. Survival, p. 10
46. Internal environment, p. 10
47. Rise, p. 15
48. Developmental processes, p. 15
49. Aging processes, p. 15
50. Negative, positive, p. 14
51. Stabilizing, p. 15
52. Stimulatory, p. 15

Applying What You Know

53. ① on diagram
54. ② on diagram
55. ③ on diagram

56.   **WORD FIND**

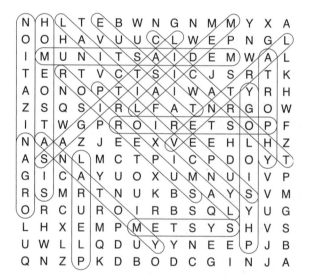

Check Your Knowledge

Multiple Choice

1. A, p. 10
2. D, p. 7
3. B, p. 10
4. D, p. 6
5. A, p. 1
6. C, p. 7
7. C, p. 4
8. A, p. 6
9. C, p. 10
10. B, p. 7
11. D, p. 10
12. B, p. 10
13. C, p. 4

14. A, p. 6
15. D, p. 6
16. C, p. 4
17. D, p. 12
18. A, p. 10
19. A, p. 10
20. C, p. 6

Matching

21. F, p. 5
22. B, p. 12
23. J, p. 6
24. G, p. 1
25. H, p. 6
26. C, p. 10
27. D, p. 10
28. I, p. 5
29. A, p. 6
30. E, p. 4

Fill in the blanks

31. Scientific method, p. 13
32. Hypothesis, p. 13
33. Experimentation, p. 13
34. Test group, p. 13
35. Control group, p. 13

Dorsal and Ventral Body Cavities

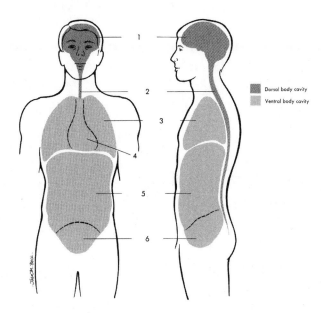

1. Cranial cavity
2. Spinal cavity
3. Thoracic cavity
4. Mediastinum
5. Abdominal cavity
6. Pelvic cavity

Directions and Planes of the Body

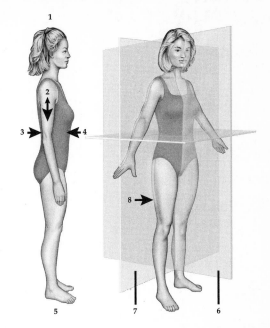

1. Superior
2. Proximal
3. Posterior (dorsal)
4. Anterior (ventral)
5. Inferior
6. Sagittal plane
7. Frontal plane
8. Lateral

Regions of the Abdomen

1. Epigastric region
2. Left hypochondriac region
3. Umbilical region
4. Left lumbar region
5. Left iliac (inguinal) region
6. Hypogastric region
7. Right iliac (inguinal) region
8. Right lumbar region
9. Right hypochondriac region

CHAPTER 2
CHEMISTRY OF LIFE

Multiple Choice

1. C, p. 22
2. B, p. 22
3. C, p. 22
4. A, p. 22
5. D, p. 22
6. C, p. 22
7. A, p. 22

True or False

8. T, p. 21
9. F (molecules), p. 22
10. F (uncharged neutrons), p. 22
11. T, p. 22
12. T, p. 22

Multiple Choice

13. C, p. 24
14. B, p. 25
15. A, p. 25
16. B, p. 25
17. A, p. 25
18. C, p. 25

Matching

19. H, p. 26
20. B, p. 26
21. E, p. 26
22. A, p. 26
23. G, p. 26
24. L, p. 26
25. J, p. 26
26. C, p. 27
27. D, p. 27
28. F, p. 27
29. K, p. 28
30. I, p. 28

Circle the Correct Answer

31. A, p. 30
32. B, p. 30
33. D, p. 33
34. B, p. 31
35. C, p. 31
36. A, p. 30
37. A, p. 30
38. B, p. 30
39. C, p. 31
40. D, p. 33

Crossword

Applying What You Know

41. Some fats can become solid at room temperature, such as the fat in butter and lard.
42. Radioactive isotopes will be used to measure Carol's thyroid activity. A diagnosis of hyperthyroidism or hypothyroidism will be based upon how rapidly or slowly the thyroid absorbs the radioactive iodine and emits radiation.

43. **WORD FIND**

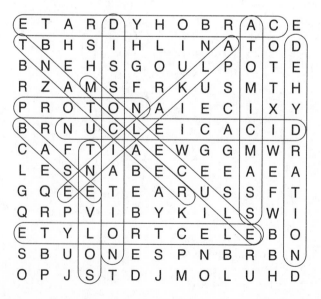

Check Your Knowledge

Fill in the Blanks

1. Biochemistry, p. 21
2. Neutrons, p. 22
3. Higher, p. 22
4. Elements; compounds, p. 22
5. Stable, p. 22
6. Ion, p. 25
7. Inorganic, p. 26
8. Dehydration synthesis, p. 26
9. Chemical equation, p. 27
10. CO_2, p. 27
11. Acids, p. 27
12. Buffers, p. 28
13. Carbohydrate, p. 30
14. Cholesterol, p. 31
15. Structural, p. 33
16. Tertiary protein structure, p. 32
17. Primary protein structure, p. 32

CHAPTER 3
CELLS AND TISSUES

Matching

Group A

1. C, p. 42
2. E, p. 42
3. A, p. 42
4. B, p. 47
5. D, p. 46

Group B

6. D, p. 46
7. E, p. 46
8. A, p. 46
9. B, p. 46
10. C, p. 46

Fill in the Blanks

11. Cholesterol, p. 42
12. Tissue typing, p. 70
13. Cilia, p. 47
14. Endoplasmic reticulum, p. 46
15. Ribosomes, p. 45
16. Mitochondria, p. 46
17. Lysosomes, p. 46
18. Golgi apparatus, p. 46
19. Centrioles, p. 46
20. Chromatin granules, p. 48
21. Rejection reaction, p. 70
22. ELISA, p. 70

Circle the Correct Answer

23. A, p. 49
24. D, p. 49
25. B, p. 49
26. D, p. 51
27. C, p. 51
28. A, p. 51
29. B, p. 51
30. C, p. 51
31. C, p. 51
32. A, p. 53
33. B, p. 53
34. A, p. 53

Circle the One That Does Not Belong

35. Uracil (RNA contains the base uracil, not DNA)
36. RNA (the others are complementary base pairings of DNA)
37. Anaphase (the others refer to genes and heredity)
38. Thymine (the others refer to RNA)
39. Interphase (the others refer to translation)
40. Prophase (the others refer to anaphase)
41. Prophase (the others refer to interphase)
42. Metaphase (the others refer to telophase)
43. Gene (the others refer to stages of cell division)

44.   Fill in the missing areas

TISSUE	LOCATION	FUNCTION
Epithelial		
1.	1.	1a. Absorption by respiratory gases between alveolar air and blood
2.	2a. Surface of lining of mouth and esophagus	2.
	2b. Surface of skin	
3.	3. Surface layer of lining of stomach, intestines, and parts of respiratory tract	3.
4. Stratified transitional	4.	4.
5.	5. Surface of lining of trachea	5.
6.	6.	6. Secretion; absorption
Connective		
1.	1. Between other tissues and organs	1.
2. Adipose	2.	2.
3.	3.	3. Flexible but strong connection
4.	4. Skeleton	4.
5.	5. Part of nasal septum, larynx, rings in trachea and bronchi, disks between vertebrae, external ear	5.
6.	6.	6. Transportation
7. Hematopoietic tissue	7.	7.
Muscle		
1.	1. Muscles that attach to bones, eyeball muscles, upper third of esophagus	1.
2. Cardiac	2.	2.
3.	3. Walls of digestive, respiratory, and genitourinary tracts; walls of blood and large lymphatic vessels; ducts of glands; intrinsic eye muscles; arrector muscles of hair	3.
Nervous		
1.	1. Brain and spinal cord, nerves	1.

Applying What You Know

45.

46. Diffusion
47. Absorption of oxygen into Ms. Bence's blood.
48. Merrily may have exceeded the 18 to 24% desirable body fat composition. Fitness depends more on the percentage and ratio of specific tissue types than the overall amount of tissue present.

49. **WORD FIND**

Crossword

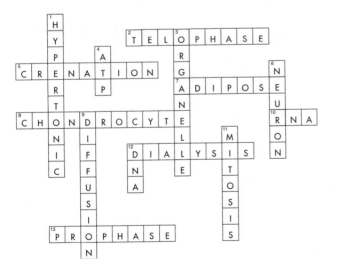

Check Your Knowledge

Multiple Choice

1. A, p. 46
2. B, p. 53
3. B, p. 48
4. A, p. 59
5. C, p. 51

6. A, p. 57
7. A, p. 68
8. B, p. 67
9. C, p. 62
10. D, p. 71

Matching

11. F, p. 68
12. G, p. 42
13. J, p. 72
14. C, p. 53
15. A, p. 58
16. B, p. 58
17. I, p. 49
18. H, p. 62
19. D, p. 46
20. E, p. 63

Cell Structure

1. Flagellum
2. Free ribosomes
3. Mitochondrion
4. Nuclear envelope
5. Nucleus
6. Nucleolus
7. Ribosomes
8. Cilia
9. Smooth endoplasmic reticulum
10. Rough endoplasmic reticulum
11. Plasma membrane
12. Lysosome
13. Cytoplasm
14. Golgi apparatus
15. Centrioles

Mitosis

1. Interphase
2. Prophase
3. Metaphase
4. Anaphase
5. Telophase
6. Daughter cells (interphase)

Tissues

1. Stratified squamous epithelium
2. Simple columnar epithelium
3. Stratified transitional epithelium
4. Adipose tissue
5. Dense fibrous connective tissue
6. Bone tissue
7. Cartilage
8. Blood
9. Skeletal muscle
10. Cardiac muscle
11. Smooth muscle
12. Nervous tissue

CHAPTER 4
ORGAN SYSTEMS OF THE BODY

Matching

Group A

1. A, p. 87
2. E, p. 87
3. D, p. 90
4. B, p. 90
5. C, p. 91

Group B

6. F, p. 91
7. E, p. 93
8. B, p. 95
9. A, p. 95
10. C, p. 94
11. D, p. 96

Circle the One That Does Not Belong

12. Mouth (the others refer to the respiratory system)
13. Rectum (the others refer to the reproductive system)
14. Pancreas (the others refer to the cardiovascular system)
15. Pineal (the others refer to the urinary system)
16. Joints (the others refer to the muscular system)
17. Pituitary (the others refer to the nervous system)
18. Tendons (the others refer to the skeletal system)
19. Appendix (the others refer to the endocrine system)
20. Thymus (the others refer to the integumentary system)
21. Trachea (the others refer to the digestive system)
22. Liver (the others refer to the lymphatic system)

Fill in the Missing Areas

SYSTEM	ORGAN	FUNCTIONS
23.	23.	23. Protection, regulation of body temperature, synthesis of chemicals and hormones, serves as a sense organ
24.	24. Bones, joints	24.
25.	25.	25. Movement, maintains body posture, produces heat
26. Nervous	26.	26.
27.	27. Pituitary, thymus, pineal, adrenal, hypothalamus, thyroid, pancreas, parathyroid, ovaries, testes	27.
28.	28.	28. Transportation, immunity, regulation of body temperature
29.	29. Lymph nodes, lymph vessels, thymus, spleen, tonsils	29.
30. Urinary	30.	30.
31.	31. Mouth, pharynx, esophagus, stomach, small and large intestine, rectum, anal canal, teeth, salivary glands, tongue, liver, gallbladder, pancreas, appendix	31.
32. Respiratory	32.	32.
33.	33a. Gonads—testes and ovaries	33.
	33b. Accessory organs (p. 107), supporting structures (p. 107)	

Fill in the Blanks

34. Nonvital organ, p. 98
35. Cochlear implants, p. 100
36. Dialysis machine, p. 101
37. Left ventricular assist systems (LVAS), p. 101
38. Organ transplantation, p. 101
39. Free-flap surgery, p. 102
40. Rejection, p. 102

Unscramble the Words

41. Heart
42. Pineal
43. Nerve
44. Esophagus
45. Nervous

Applying What You Know

46. (a) Endocrinology (endocrine system)
    (b) Gynecology (reproductive system)
47. The skin protects the underlying tissue against invasion by harmful bacteria. With a large percentage of Brian's skin destroyed, he was vulnerable to bacteria, and so he was placed in the cleanest environment possible—isolation. Jenny is required to wear special attire so that the risk of a visitor bringing bacteria to the patient is reduced.
48. Free-flap surgery may be considered as an option. A breast can be formed from skin and muscle taken from other parts of Sheila's body.

49. **WORD FIND**

Crossword

Check Your Knowledge

Multiple Choice

1. D, p. 95
2. C, p. 91 and 96
3. C, p. 95
4. B, p. 90
5. D, p. 87
6. A, p. 95
7. B, p. 105
8. A, p. 87
9. A, p. 93
10. C, p. 85

Matching

11. C, p. 87
12. D, p. 91
13. H, p. 93
14. G, p. 96
15. B, p. 95
16. F, p. 95
17. I, p. 96
18. E, p. 94
19. J, p. 90
20. A, p. 91

CHAPTER 5
MECHANISMS OF DISEASE

Matching

Group A

1. B, p. 111
2. E, p. 112
3. A, p. 112
4. C, p. 112
5. D, p. 112

Group B

6. C, p. 112
7. A, p. 112
8. D, p. 112
9. B, p. 112
10. E, p. 112

Fill in the Blanks

11. Pathophysiology, p. 113
12. Homeostasis, p. 113
13. Mutated, p. 114
14. Parasite, p. 114
15. Neoplasms, p. 114
16. Self-immunity, p. 114
17. Risk factors, p. 115
18. Centers for Disease Control and Prevention, p. 115
19. Psychogenic, p. 115
20. Secondary, p. 115

Multiple Choice

21. C, p. 116
22. A, p. 117
23. B, p. 118
24. C, p. 118
25. D, p. 118
26. B, p. 120
27. D, p. 122
28. D, p. 123
29. B, p. 125
30. C, p. 125
31. E, p. 125
32. B, p. 126

Circle the Correct Answer

33. Slowly, p. 126
34. Are not, p. 126
35. Papilloma, p. 127
36. Sarcoma, p. 128

37. Anaplasia, p. 129
38. Oncologist, p. 130
39. Biopsy, p. 131
40. Staging, p. 131
41. Appetite, p. 131

Warning Signs of Cancer, p. 130

42. Sores that do not heal
43. Unusual bleeding
44. A change in a wart or mole
45. A lump or thickening in any tissue
46. Persistent hoarseness or cough
47. Chronic indigestion
48. A change in bowel or bladder function
49. Bone pain that wakes the person at night and is located only on one side

True or False

50. T
51. F (slowly), p. 136
52. F (white), p. 136
53. T
54. F (regeneration), p. 137
55. T
56. T

Unscramble the Words

57. Fungi
58. Oncogene
59. Edema
60. Spore
61. Grading

Applying What You Know

62. No. Trent most likely has a common cold.
63. Pinworm
64. Disinfection
65. A "gene pool" indicates the "risk" of inheriting a disease-causing gene specific to members of a certain ethnic group. The knowledge of a "gene pool" can alert you to early detection of disease.
66. Bill is considering a "high risk" profession because of the paramedic's frequent exposure to body fluids. Hepatitis B is transmitted by body fluids and, therefore, vaccination is recommended.

67.   WORD FIND

9.   D, p. 116
10.   A, p. 123

Matching

11.   C, p. 112
12.   D, p. 127
13.   B, p. 118
14.   J, p. 120
15.   G, p. 112
16.   I, p. 137
17.   E, p. 123
18.   A, p. 111
19.   F, p. 126
20.   H, p. 123

Crossword

Check Your Knowledge

Multiple Choice

1.   B, p. 112
2.   D, p. 112
3.   A, p. 126
4.   D, p. 112
5.   A, p. 119
6.   D, p. 112
7.   C, p. 113
8.   B, p. 131

Major Groups of Pathogenic Bacteria

1.   Bacilli (rods)
2.   Cocci (spheres)
3.   Curved rods
4.   Small bacteria

Major Groups of Pathogenic Protozoa

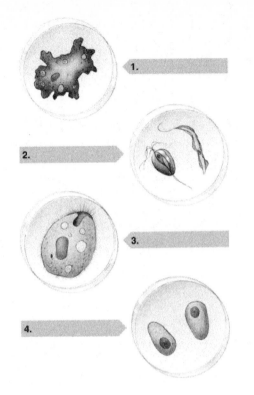

1.   Amoebas
2.   Flagellates
3.   Ciliates
4.   Sporozoa

Examples of Pathogenic Animals

1.   Nematodes
2.   Platyhelminths
3.   Arthropods

Major Groups of Pathogenic Fungi

1.   Yeasts
2.   Molds

CHAPTER 6
THE INTEGUMENTARY SYSTEM AND BODY MEMBRANES

Select the Best Answer

1.   B, p. 148
2.   D, p. 150
3.   C, p. 149
4.   A, p. 148
5.   B, p. 148
6.   D, p. 150
7.   C, p. 149
8.   C, p. 148

Matching

Group A

9.   D, p. 150
10.   A, p. 150
11.   B, p. 150
12.   C, p. 150
13.   E, p. 150

Group B

14.   A, p. 152
15.   D, p. 152
16.   E, p. 152
17.   C, p. 158
18.   B, p. 152

Select the Best Answer

19.   A, p. 150
20.   B, p. 161

21. B, p. 158
22. A, p. 158
23. A, p. 152
24. B, p. 158
25. B, p. 159
26. B, p. 163
27. B, p. 162
28. A, p. 152

Fill in the Blanks

29. Protection, temperature regulation, and sense organ activity, p. 163
30. Melanin, p. 152
31. Lanugo, p. 159
32. Hair papillae, p. 159
33. Alopecia, p. 160
34. Arrector pili, p. 160
35. Strawberry hemangioma, p. 159
36. Eccrine, p. 162
37. Apocrine, p. 162
38. Sebum, p. 163

Circle the Correct Answer

39. Will not, p. 165
40. Will, p. 165
41. Will not, p. 165
42. 11, p. 167
43. Third-, p. 165

Circle the Correct Answer

44. B, p. 164
45. A, p. 164
46. D, p. 154
47. D, p. 157
48. A, p. 163
49. D, p. 168
50. C, p. 168
51. A, p. 170

Unscramble the Words

52. Epidermis
53. Keratin
54. Hair
55. Lanugo
56. Dehydration
57. Third Degree

Applying What You Know

58. 46
59. Pleurisy
60. Sunbathing. Mrs. Collins cannot repair UV damage and thus is very prone to skin cancer.
61. Fingerprints

62. **WORD FIND**

Crossword

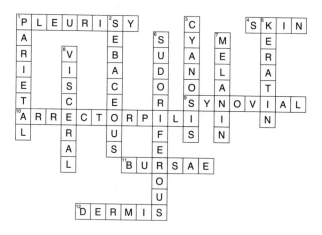

Check Your Knowledge

Multiple Choice

1. A, p. 148
2. B, p. 150
3. A, p. 160
4. D, p. 162
5. B, p. 152
6. D, p. 165
7. B, p. 163
8. B, p. 152
9. C, p. 161
10. B, p. 163

Matching

11. C, p. 152
12. D, p. 148
13. B, p. 161

14. G, p. 163
15. I, p. 152
16. H, p. 159
17. J, p. 161
18. E, p. 150
19. A, p. 158
20. F, p. 162

Completion

21. H, p. 163
22. A, p. 163
23. B, p. 162
24. F, p. 165
25. I, p. 159
26. E, p. 150
27. G, p. 148
28. D, p. 148
29. J, p. 161
30. C, p. 148

Longitudinal Section of the Skin

1. Opening of sweat ducts
2. Epidermis
3. Dermis
4. Subcutaneous fatty tissue (hypodermis)
5. Sweat gland
6. Arrector pili muscle
7. Pacinian corpuscle
8. Cutaneous nerve
9. Papilla of hair
10. Hair follicle
11. Sebaceous (oil) gland
12. Meissner's corpuscle
13. Dermal papilla
14. Stratum germinativum
15. Stratum corneum
16. Hair shaft

Rule of Nines

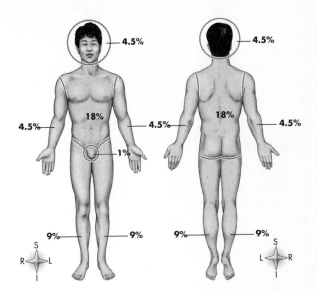

CHAPTER 7
THE SKELETAL SYSTEM

Fill in the Blanks

1. Four, p. 182
2. Medullary cavity, p. 182
3. Articular cartilage, p. 182
4. Endosteum, p. 182
5. Hematopoiesis, p. 182
6. Red bone marrow, p. 182
7. Periosteum, p. 183
8. Long, short, flat, and irregular, p. 182
9. Calcium, p. 182
10. Move, p. 182

Matching

Group A

11. D, p. 183
12. B, p. 183
13. E, p. 183
14. A, p. 184
15. C, p. 184

Group B

16. D, p. 183
17. A, p. 183
18. E, p. 183
19. B, p. 184
20. C, p. 183

True or False

21. T

22. F (Epiphyses, not diaphyses), p. 185
23. F (Osteoblasts, not osteoclasts), p. 185
24. T
25. T
26. F (Juvenile, not adult), p. 186
27. F (Diaphysis, not articulation), p. 185
28. T
29. F (Ceases, not begins), p. 186
30. T

Multiple Choice

31. A, p. 187
32. D, p. 190
33. A, p. 194
34. D, p. 196
35. C, p. 197
36. C, p. 202
37. D, p. 197
38. D, p. 200
39. A, p. 202
40. B, p. 190
41. A, p. 194
42. B, p. 200
43. B, p. 196
44. B, p. 197
45. C, p. 197
46. A, p. 202
47. D, p. 190
48. C, p. 194
49. C, p. 190

Circle the One That Does Not Belong

50. Coxal (all others refer to the spine)
51. Axial (all others refer to the appendicular skeleton)
52. Maxilla (all others refer to the cranial bones)
53. Ribs (all others refer to the shoulder girdle)
54. Vomer (all others refer to the bones of the middle ear)
55. Ulna (all others refer to the coxal bone)
56. Ethmoid (all others refer to the hand and wrist)
57. Nasal (all others refer to cranial bones)
58. Anvil (all others refer to the cervical vertebra)

Choose the Correct Answer

59. A, p. 205
60. B, p. 205
61. B, p. 205
62. A, p. 204
63. B, p. 205

Matching

64. C, p. 190

65. G, p. 196
66. J, L, M, and K, p. 203
67. N, p. 203
68. I, p. 200
69. A, p. 190
70. P, p. 203
71. D, B, p. 190
72. F, p. 190
73. H, Q, p. 200
74. O, T, p. 203
75. R, p. 190
76. S, E, p. 190

Circle the Correct Answer

77. Diarthroses, p. 205
78. Synarthrotic, p. 205
79. Diarthrotic, p. 206
80. Ligaments, p. 206
81. Articular cartilage, p. 206
82. Least movable, p. 208
83. Largest, p. 209
84. 2, p. 208
85. Mobility, p. 208
86. Pivot, p. 208

Fill in the Blanks

87. Arthroscopy, p. 217
88. Osteosarcoma, p. 212
89. Osteoporosis, p. 213
90. Osteomalacia, p. 213
91. Paget's disease, p. 213
92. Osteomyelitis, p. 214
93. Simple fractures, p. 215
94. Comminuted fractures, p. 215
95. Osteoarthritis or degenerative joint disease (DJD), p. 215
96. Rheumatoid arthritis, gouty arthritis, and infectious arthritis, p. 218
97. Lyme disease, p. 219

Unscramble the Bones

98. Vertebrae
99. Pubis
100. Scapula
101. Mandible
102. Phalanges
103. Pelvic girdle

Applying What You Know

104. The bones are responsible for the majority of our blood cell formation. Her disease condition might be inhibiting the production of blood cells.

105. Epiphyseal cartilage is present only while a child is still growing. It becomes bone in adulthood. It is particularly vulnerable to fractures in childhood and preadolescence.
106. Osteoporosis
107. Slipped or herniated disk

108. **WORD FIND**

Crossword

Check Your Knowledge

Multiple Choice

1. A, p. 196
2. C, p. 197

3. A, p. 182
4. C, p. 204
5. C, p. 194
6. D, p. 208
7. C, p. 187
8. C, p. 190
9. D, p. 185
10. A, p. 205

Matching

11. G, p. 206
12. B, p. 183
13. I, p. 205
14. J, p. 190
15. E, p. 203
16. H, p. 184
17. A, p. 183
18. C, p. 190
19. F, p. 203
20. D, p. 183

Longitudinal Section of Long Bone

1. Articular cartilage
2. Epiphyseal plate
3. Spongy bone
4. Red marrow cavities
5. Compact bone
6. Yellow marrow
7. Periosteum
8. Endosteum
9. Medullary cavity
10. Epiphysis
11. Diaphysis

Anterior View of Skeleton

1. Orbit
2. Mandible
3. Sternum
4. Xiphoid process
5. Costal cartilage
6. Coxal
7. Ilium
8. Pubis
9. Ischium
10. Frontal
11. Nasal
12. Maxilla
13. Clavicle
14. Ribs
15. Humerus
16. Vertebral column
17. Ulna
18. Radius
19. Sacrum
20. Coccyx
21. Carpals
22. Metacarpals
23. Phalanges
24. Femur
25. Patella
26. Tibia
27. Fibula
28. Tarsals
29. Metatarsals
30. Phalanges

Posterior View of Skeleton

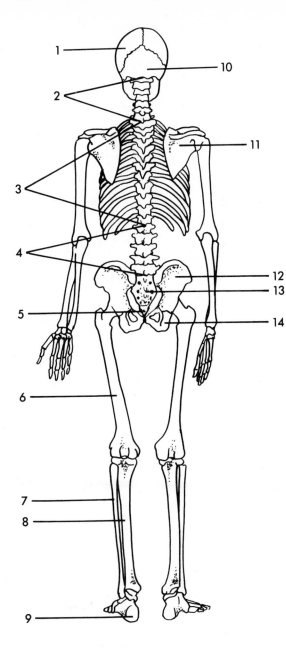

Skull Viewed from the Right Side

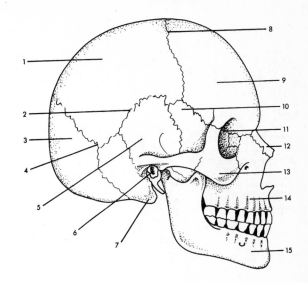

1.   Parietal bone
2.   Squamous suture
3.   Occipital bone
4.   Lambdoidal suture
5.   Temporal bone
6.   External auditory canal
7.   Mastoid process
8.   Coronal suture
9.   Frontal bone
10.   Sphenoid bone
11.   Ethmoid bone
12.   Nasal bone
13.   Zygomatic bone
14.   Maxilla
15.   Mandible

1.   Parietal
2.   Cervical vertebrae
3.   Thoracic vertebrae
4.   Lumbar vertebrae
5.   Coccyx
6.   Femur
7.   Fibula
8.   Tibia
9.   Calcaneus
10.   Occipital
11.   Scapula
12.   Coxal (hip) bone
13.   Sacrum
14.   Ischium

Skull Viewed from the Front

1. Sphenoid bone
2. Ethmoid bone
3. Lacrimal bone
4. Zygomatic bone
5. Vomer
6. Frontal bone
7. Parietal bone
8. Nasal bone
9. Inferior concha
10. Maxilla
11. Mandible

Diarthrotic Joint

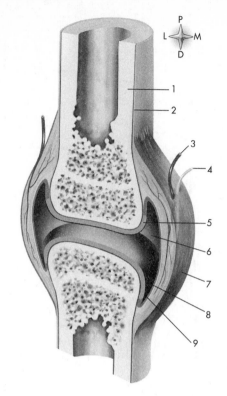

1. Bone
2. Periosteum
3. Blood vessel
4. Nerve
5. Articular cartilage
6. Joint cavity
7. Joint capsule
8. Bursa
9. Synovial membrane

CHAPTER 8
THE MUSCULAR SYSTEM

Select the Correct Term

1. A, p. 230
2. B, p. 230
3. C, p. 231
4. C, p. 230
5. A, p. 230
6. B, p. 230
7. C, (may also be B), p. 231 and Chapter 3
8. A, p. 230
9. C, p. 231
10. C, p. 231

Matching

Group A

11. D, p. 231
12. B, p. 231
13. A, p. 231
14. E, p. 231
15. C, p. 231

Group B

16. E, p. 231
17. C, p. 231
18. B, p. 231
19. A, p. 231
20. D, p. 231

Fill in the Blanks

21. Pulling, p. 233
22. Insertion, p. 233
23. Insertion, origin, p. 233
24. Prime mover, p. 233
25. Antagonists, p. 233
26. Synergist, p. 233
27. Tonic contraction, p. 234
28. Muscle tone, p. 234
29. Hypothermia, p. 234
30. ATP, p. 234

True or False

31. F (Neuromuscular junction), p. 235
32. T
33. T
34. F (Oxygen debt), p. 234
35. F ("All or none"), p. 235
36. F (Lactic acid), p. 234
37. T
38. T
39. F (Skeletal muscles), p. 234
40. T

Multiple Choice

41. A, p. 236
42. B, p. 236
43. B, p. 237
44. C, p. 238
45. D, p. 238
46. A, p. 235
47. B, p. 236
48. C, p. 236
49. B, p. 238
50. D, p. 238

Matching

51. C, p. 231
52. F, p. 242; A and D, p. 249
53. F, p. 242 and B, p. 249
54. A, p. 241
55. C, p. 249
56. B, p. 249 and F, p. 242
57. A, p. 241
58. A and D, p. 241
59. B, p. 241
60. B, p. 241
61. A and E, p. 241
62. B, p. 241
63. D, p. 241

Multiple Choice

64. A, p. 246
65. D, p. 247
66. C, p. 247
67. A, p. 247
68. D, p. 247
69. C, p. 247

Circle the Correct Answer

70. Myalgia, p. 249
71. Myoglobin, p. 250
72. Poliomyelitis, p. 251
73. Muscular dystrophy, p. 251
74. Myasthenia gravis, p. 251

Applying What You Know

75. Bursitis
76. Deltoid area
77. Tendon

78. **WORD FIND**

Crossword

Muscles—Anterior View

Check Your Knowledge

Multiple Choice

1. D, p. 235
2. A, p. 247
3. C, p. 233
4. B, p. 245
5. A, p. 235
6. B, p. 234
7. D, p. 235
8. A, p. 238
9. A, p. 250
10. C, p. 231

True or False

11. T, p. 247
12. T, p. 236
13. F (Pronation), p. 247
14. F (Hypertrophy), p. 238
15. T, p. 236
16. T, p. 234
17. T, p. 231
18. F (Hypothermia), p. 234
19. T, p. 236
20. F (Flexion), p. 246

1. Sternocleidomastoid
2. Trapezius
3. Pectoralis major
4. Rectus abdominis
5. External abdominal oblique
6. Iliopsoas
7. Quadriceps group
8. Tibialis anterior
9. Peroneus longus
10. Peroneus brevis
11. Soleus
12. Gastrocnemius
13. Sartorius
14. Adductor group
15. Brachialis
16. Biceps brachii
17. Deltoid
18. Facial muscles

Muscles—Posterior View

1. Trapezius
2. External abdominal oblique
3. Gluteus maximus
4. Adductor magnus
5. Soleus
6. Peroneus brevis
7. Peroneus longus
8. Gastrocnemius
9. Hamstring group
10. Latissimus dorsi
11. Triceps brachii
12. Deltoid
13. Sternocleidomastoid

CHAPTER 9
THE NERVOUS SYSTEM

Matching

Group A

1. B, p. 262
2. C, p. 262
3. D, p. 262
4. A, p. 262

Group B

5. B, p. 262
6. D, p. 262
7. C, p. 262
8. A, p. 262
9. F, p. 267
10. E, p. 267

Select the Best Choice

11. A, p. 262
12. B, p. 263
13. B, p. 265
14. A, p. 262
15. A, p. 262
16. B, p. 265
17. B, p. 265
18. A, p. 262
19. B, p. 265
20. A, p. 262

Fill in the Blanks

21. Two-neuron arc, p. 267
22. Sensory neurons, interneurons, and motor neurons, p. 267
23. Receptors, p. 267
24. Synapse, p. 268
25. Reflex, p. 269
26. Withdrawal reflex, p. 269
27. Ganglion, p. 267
28. Interneurons, p. 269
29. "Knee jerk," p. 269
30. Gray matter, p. 269

Circle the Correct Answer

31. Do not, p. 270
32. Increases, p. 270
33. Excess, p. 270
34. Postsynaptic, p. 270
35. Presynaptic, p. 270
36. Neurotransmitter, p. 272
37. Communicate, p. 270
38. Specifically, p. 272
39. Sleep, p. 273
40. Pain, p. 273

Multiple Choice

41. E, p. 275
42. D, p. 275
43. A, p. 277
44. E, p. 277
45. E, p. 277
46. D, p. 277
47. B, p. 278
48. E, p. 278
49. B, p. 278
50. D, p. 278
51. D, p. 278
52. B, p. 278
53. A, p. 278
54. D, p. 278
55. C, p. 278

Select the Best Choice

56. H, p. 278
57. D, p. 280
58. E, p. 080
59. C, p. 281
60. J, p. 281
61. A, p. 281

62. B, p. 281
63. F, p. 281
64. I, p. 280
65. G, p. 282

True or False

66. F (17 to 18 inches), p. 282
67. F (Bottom of the first lumbar vertebra), p. 282
68. F (Lumbar punctures), p. 287
69. F (Spinal tracts), p. 282
70. T
71. F (One general function), p. 283
72. F (Anesthesia), p. 284

Circle the One That Does Not Belong

73. Ventricles (all others refer to meninges)
74. CSF (all others refer to the arachnoid)
75. Pia mater (all others refer to the cerebrospinal fluid)
76. Choroid plexus (all others refer to the dura mater)
77. Brain tumor (all others refer to a lumbar puncture)

Cranial Nerves

78. Fill in the missing areas on the chart below.

Nerve		Conduct Impulses	Function
I	Olfactory		
II			Vision
III		From brain to eye muscles	
IV	Trochlear		
V			Sensations of face, scalp, and teeth, chewing movements
VI		From brain to external eye muscles	
VII			Sense of taste; Contraction of muscles of facial expression
VIII	Vestibulocochlear		
IX		From throat and taste buds of tongue to brain; also from brain to throat muscles and salivary glands	
X	Vagus		
XI			Shoulder movements; turning movements of head
XII	Hypoglossal		

Select the Best Choice

79. A, p. 289
80. B, p. 291
81. A, p. 289
82. B, p. 292
83. B, p. 290
84. A, p. 289
85. B, p. 290
86. B, p. 290

Matching

87. D, p. 292
88. E, p. 294
89. F, p. 295
90. B, p. 295
91. A, p. 294
92. C, p. 294

Multiple Choice

93. C, p. 295
94. B, p. 295
95. B, p. 296
96. D, p. 295
97. A, p. 295
98. A, p. 297

Choose the Correct Answer

99. B, p. 297
100. A, p. 297
101. A, p. 297
102. B, p. 297
103. A, p. 297
104. B, p. 297
105. A, p. 297
106. A, p. 297
107. B, p. 297
108. B, p. 297

Fill in the Blanks

109. Acetylcholine, p. 297
110. Adrenergic fibers, p. 297
111. Cholinergic fibers, p. 297
112. Homeostasis, p. 298
113. Heart rate, p. 298
114. Decreased, p. 299
115. Neuroblastoma, p. 299

Unscramble the Words

116. Neurons
117. Synapse
118. Autonomic
119. Smooth muscle
120. Sympathetic

Applying What You Know

121. Right
122. Hydrocephalus
123. Sympathetic
124. Parasympathetic
125. Sympathetic. No, the digestive process is not active during sympathetic control. Bill may experience nausea, vomiting, or discomfort because of this factor. See p. 294.

126. **WORD FIND**

Crossword

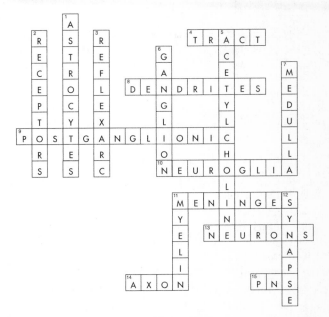

Check Your Knowledge

Multiple Choice

1. D, p. 262
2. B, p. 286
3. A, p. 285
4. B, p. 277
5. A, p. 297
6. D, p. 297
7. D, p. 262
8. C, p. 270
9. C, p. 283
10. D, p. 292

Matching

11. C, p. 282
12. A, p. 262
13. J, p. 275
14. H, p. 272
15. B, p. 269
16. I, p. 291
17. F, p. 263
18. E, p. 277
19. D, p. 289
20. G, p. 278

Neuron

1. Dendrites
2. Cell body
3. Nucleus
4. Axon
5. Schwann cell
6. Myelin
7. Mitochondrion

Cranial Nerves

1. Olfactory nerve (I)
2. Trigeminal nerve (V)
3. Glossopharyngeal nerve (IX)
4. Hypoglossal nerve (XII)
5. Accessory nerve (XI)
6. Vagus nerve (X)
7. Vestibulocochlear nerve (VIII)
8. Facial nerve (VII)
9. Abducens nerve (VI)
10. Oculomotor nerve (III)
11. Optic nerve (II)
12. Trochlear nerve (IV)

Sagittal Section of the Central Nervous System

1. Skull
2. Pineal gland
3. Cerebellum
4. Midbrain
5. Spinal cord
6. Medulla
7. Reticular formation
8. Pons
9. Pituitary gland
10. Hypothalamus
11. Cerebral cortex
12. Thalamus
13. Corpus callosum

The Cerebrum

1. Occipital lobe
2. Temporal lobe
3. Lateral fissure
4. Frontal lobe
5. Central Sulcus
6. Parietal lobe

Neuron Pathways

1. Somatic motor neuron's axon
2. Cell body of somatic motor neuron
3. Cell body of preganglionic neuron
4. Collateral ganglion
5. Postganglionic neuron's axon
6. Preganglionic sympathetic neuron's axon

CHAPTER 10
THE SENSES

Matching

1. D, p. 311
2. B, p. 311
3. A, p. 314
4. E, p. 313
5. C, p. 314

Multiple Choice

6. C, p. 315
7. E, p. 316
8. B, p. 315
9. C, p. 316
10. E, p. 316
11. D, p. 316
12. A, p. 316
13. B, p. 316
14. C, p. 318
15. B, p. 318
16. D, p. 318
17. A, p. 314
18. D, p. 316

Select the Best Answer

19. C, p. 320
20. E, p. 320
21. F, p. 322
22. A, p. 322

23. J, p. 320
24. B, p. 324
25. H, p. 320
26. G, p. 324
27. I, p. 326
28. D, p. 324

Select the Best Answer

29. B, p. 329
30. C, p. 329
31. B, p. 329
32. A, p. 327
33. C, p. 329
34. A, p. 326
35. C, p. 329
36. B, p. 329
37. A, p. 327
38. C, p. 331

Fill in the Blanks

39. Auricle; external auditory canal, p. 326
40. Eardrum, p. 327
41. Ossicles, p. 329
42. Oval window, p. 329
43. Otitis media, p. 329
44. Vestibule, p. 329
45. Mechanoreceptors, p. 329
46. Crista ampullaris, p. 329

Select the Best Answer

47. C, p. 332
48. A, p. 332
49. D, p. 332
50. E, p. 332
51. B, p. 332
52. F, p. 332

Circle the Correct Answer

53. Papillae, p. 332
54. Cranial, p. 332
55. Mucus, p. 332
56. Memory, p. 334
57. Chemoreceptors, p. 332

Unscramble the Words

58. Auricle
59. Sclera
60. Papilla
61. Conjunctiva
62. Pupils

Applying What You Know

63. External otitis

64. Cataracts
65. The eustachian tube connects the throat to the middle ear and provides a perfect pathway for the spread of infection.
66. Olfactory

67. **WORD FIND**

Crossword

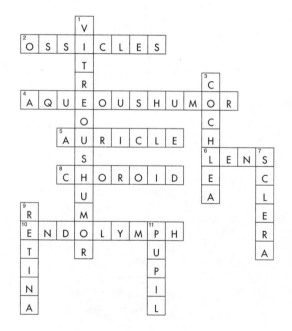

Check Your Knowledge

Multiple Choice

1. A, p. 329
2. B, p. 331
3. A, p. 332
4. C, p. 323

5. B, p. 315
6. B, p. 313
7. D, p. 318
8. B, p. 316
9. D, p. 332
10. A, p. 326

True or False

11. T, p. 327
12. F (Aqueous humor), p. 318
13. T, p. 320
14. F (Semicircular canals), p. 329
15. T, p. 320
16. T, p. 316
17. T, p. 316
18. T, p. 316
19. T, p. 314
20. T, p. 314

Eye

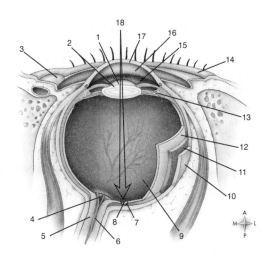

1. Lens
2. Pupil
3. Lacrimal caruncle
4. Optic disc
5. Optic nerve
6. Central artery and vein
7. Macula lutea
8. Fovea
9. Posterior chamber
10. Sclera
11. Choroid
12. Retina
13. Ciliary body
14. Lower lid
15. Iris
16. Anterior chamber
17. Cornea
18. Visual axis

Ear

1. Auricle (pinna)
2. Temporal bone
3. Malleus
4. Incus
5. Stapes
6. Semicircular canals
7. Oval window
8. Vestibular nerve
9. Cochlear nerve
10. Vestibule
11. Cochlea
12. Auditory tube
13. Tympanic membrane
14. External auditory meatus

CHAPTER 11
THE ENDOCRINE SYSTEM

Matching

Group A

1. D, p. 344
2. C, p. 344
3. E, p. 344
4. A, p. 344
5. B, p. 344

Group B

6. E, p. 348
7. C, p. 351
8. A, p. 348
9. D, p. 343
10. B, p. 344

Fill in the Blanks

11. Second messenger, p. 347
12. Protein, p. 347
13. First messenger, p. 347
14. Target organs, p. 347
15. Cyclic AMP, p. 348
16. Target cells, p. 348
17. Steroid abuse, p. 350

Multiple Choice

18. B, p. 352
19. E, p. 352
20. D, p. 352
21. D, p. 352
22. A, p. 353
23. C, p. 352
24. C, p. 354
25. B, p. 352
26. A, p. 352
27. A, p. 352
28. D, p. 354
29. B, p. 354
30. A, p. 355
31. C, p. 355
32. C, p. 355

Select the Best Answer

33. A, p. 352
34. B, p. 352
35. B, p. 355
36. C, p. 355
37. A, p. 353
38. C, p. 355
39. A, p. 352
40. A, p. 352
41. A, p. 353
42. C, p. 355

Circle the Correct Answer

43. Below, p. 355
44. Calcitonin, p. 355
45. Iodine, p. 355
46. Do not, p. 355
47. Thyroid, p. 356
48. Decreases, p. 356
49. Hypothyroidism, p. 357
50. Cretinism, p. 357
51. PTH, p. 358
52. Increase, p. 358

Fill in the Blanks

53. Adrenal cortex; adrenal medulla, p. 358
54. Corticoids, p. 360

55. Mineralocorticoids, p. 360
56. Glucocorticoids, p. 360
57. Sex hormones, p. 360
58. Gluconeogenesis, p. 360
59. Blood pressure, p. 360
60. Epinephrine; norepinephrine, p. 361
61. Stress, p. 361
62. Virilizing, p. 362

Select the Best Response

63. A, p. 363
64. A, p. 360
65. B, p. 361
66. A, p. 362
67. B, p. 361
68. A, p. 360
69. A, p. 359

Circle the Term That Does Not Belong

70. Beta cells (all others refer to glucagon)
71. Glucagon (all others refer to insulin)
72. Thymosin (all others refer to female sex glands)
73. Chorion (all others refer to male sex glands)
74. Aldosterone (all others refer to the thymus gland)
75. ACTH (all others refer to the placenta)
76. Semen (all others refer to the pineal gland)

Matching

Group A

77. E, p. 363
78. C, p. 363
79. B, p. 366
80. D, p. 366
81. A, p. 366

Group B

82. E, p. 367
83. A, p. 367
84. B, p. 367
85. C, p. 366
86. D, p. 367

Unscramble the Words

87. Corticoids
88. Diuresis
89. Glucocorticoids
90. Steroids
91. Stress

Applying What You Know

92. She was pregnant.
93. The inner zone reticularis of the adrenal cortex
94. Oxytocin

95. **WORD FIND**

Crossword

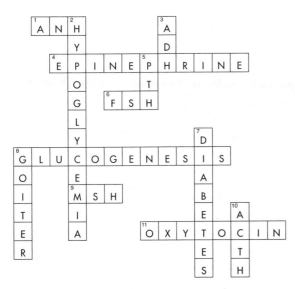

Check Your Knowledge

Multiple Choice

1. A, p. 360
2. C, p. 355
3. D, p. 357
4. B, p. 353
5. D, p. 366
6. D, p. 354
7. B, p. 367

8. D, p. 360
9. D, p. 363
10. B, p. 351

Matching

11. J, p. 357
12. G, p. 352
13. H, p. 363
14. I, p. 354
15. B, p. 355
16. F, p. 367
17. A, p. 362
18. D, p. 355
19. E, p. 353
20. C, p. 357

Endocrine Glands

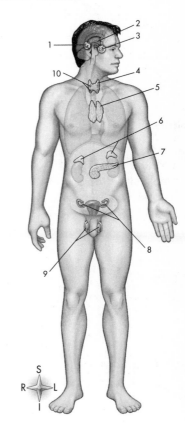

1. Pineal
2. Hypothalamus
3. Pituitary
4. Thyroid
5. Thymus
6. Adrenals
7. Pancreas (islets)
8. Ovaries (female)
9. Testes (male)
10. Parathyroids

CHAPTER 12
BLOOD

Multiple Choice

1.   E, p. 380
2.   D, p. 380
3.   D, p. 380
4.   A, p. 381
5.   D, p. 381

Fill in the Blank Areas

6.

Blood Type	Antigen Present in RBC	Antibody Present in Plasma
A	A	Anti-B
B	B	Anti-A
AB	A, B	None
O	None	Anti-A, Anti-B

Fill in the Blanks

7.   Antigen, p. 381
8.   Antibody, p. 381
9.   Agglutinate, p. 381
10.   Erythroblastosis fetalis, p. 382
11.   Rhesus monkey, p. 382
12.   Type O, p. 382
13.   Type AB, p. 382

Multiple Choice

14.   B, p. 384
15.   C, p. 384
16.   A, p. 389
17.   B, p. 387
18.   D, p. 384
19.   C, p. 387
20.   D, p. 389
21.   A, p. 390
22.   B, p. 385
23.   B, p. 387
24.   B, p. 384
25.   E, p. 386
26.   B, p. 385
27.   C, p. 385
28.   D, p. 385
29.   D, p. 387
30.   D, p. 387
31.   B, p. 393
32.   D, p. 386
33.   B, p. 393

34.   C, p. 394
35.   B, p. 394
36.   A, p. 399
37.   E, p. 399
38.   B, p. 388
39.   C, p. 390
40.   A, p. 399
41.   C, p. 393

Applying What You Know

42.   No. If Mrs. Florez were a negative Rh factor and her husband were a positive Rh factor, it would set up the strong possibility of erythroblastosis fetalis.
43.   Both procedures assist the clotting process.
44.   Anemia

45.   **WORD FIND**

Crossword

Check Your Knowledge

Multiple Choice

1. B, p. 395
2. B, p. 388
3. A, p. 385
4. A, p. 383
5. D, p. 382
6. A, p. 393
7. A, p. 399
8. D, p. 382
9. C, p. 386
10. B, p. 397

Matching

11. D, p. 394
12. F, p. 388
13. H, p. 382
14. A, p. 393
15. G, p. 395
16. C, p. 397
17. B, p. 382
18. E, p. 382
19. I, p. 385
20. J, p. 393

Human Blood Cells

1. Red blood cells
2. Platelets
3. Basophil
4. Neutrophil
5. Eosinophil
6. Lymphocyte
7. Monocyte

Blood Typing

Recipient's blood		Reactions with donor's blood			
RBC antigens	Plasma antibodies	Donor type O	Donor type A	Donor type B	Donor type AB
None (Type O)	Anti-A Anti-B				
A (Type A)	Anti-B				
B (Type B)	Anti-A				
AB (Type AB)	(none)				

Normal blood   Agglutinated blood

CHAPTER 13
THE HEART AND HEART DISEASE

Fill in the Blanks

1. Circulatory system, p. 411
2. Apex, p. 413
3. Interatrial septum, p. 413
4. Atria, p. 413
5. Ventricles, p. 413
6. Myocardium, p. 413
7. Endocarditis, p. 413
8. Bicuspid or mitral and tricuspid, p. 415
9. Visceral pericardium or epicardium, p. 413
10. Parietal pericardium, p. 413
11. Pericarditis, p. 413
12. Semilunar valves, p. 415
13. Mitral valve prolapse, p. 415
14. Rheumatic heart disease, p. 415

Select the Best Answer

15. F, p. 418
16. C, p. 419
17. D, p. 419
18. A, p. 417
19. B, p. 418
20. G, p. 420
21. E, p. 420
22. H, p. 420
23. J, p. 417
24. I, p. 420

Circle the Correct Answer

25. B, p. 420
26. C p. 421

27. A, p. 421
28. C, p. 424
29. A, p. 421
30. D, p. 421
31. C, p. 425
32. A, p. 425
33. B, p. 426
34. C, p. 426
35. A, p. 425
36. D, p. 425

Applying What You Know

37. Coronary bypass surgery
38. Artificial pacemaker
39. The endocardial lining can become rough and abrasive to red blood cells passing over its surface. As a result, a fatal blood clot may be formed.
40. 3   Tricuspid valve
    6   Pulmonary arteries
    9   Bicuspid valve
    1   Vena cavae
    4   Right ventricle
    12 Aorta
    7   Pulmonary veins
    5   Pulmonary semilunar valve
    10 Left ventricle
    2   Right atrium
    8   Left atrium
    11 Aortic semilunar valve

41. **WORD FIND**

Crossword

Check Your Knowledge

Multiple Choice

1. C, p. 417
2. D, p. 421
3. C, p. 424
4. D, p. 413
5. C, p. 413
6. B, p. 413
7. D, p. 415
8. A, p. 421
9. C, p. 424
10. D, p. 426

Matching

11. F, p. 419
12. G, p. 421
13. H, p. 415
14. I, p. 418
15. J, p. 415
16. B, p. 415
17. C, p. 413
18. A, p. 421
19. D, p. 421
20. E, p. 420

The Heart

Conduction System of the Heart

1. Left common carotid artery
2. Left subclavian artery
3. Arch of aorta
4. Left pulmonary artery
5. Left atrium
6. Left pulmonary veins
7. Great cardiac vein
8. Branches of left coronary artery and cardiac vein
9. Left ventricle
10. Apex
11. Right ventricle
12. Right atrium
13. Right coronary artery and cardiac vein
14. Right pulmonary veins
15. Ascending aorta
16. Right pulmonary artery
17. Superior vena cava
18. Brachiocephalic trunk

1. Aorta
2. Pulmonary artery
3. Pulmonary veins
4. Mitral valve (bicuspid)
5. Purkinje fibers
6. Right and left branches of AV bundle (bundle of His)
7. Left ventricle
8. Inferior vena cava
9. Right ventricle
10. Tricuspid valve
11. Atrioventricular (AV) node
12. Sinoatrial (SA) node (pacemaker)
13. Superior vena cava

Normal ECG Deflections

1.   Atrial depolarization
2.   Ventricular depolarization
3.   Ventricular repolarization

CHAPTER 14
THE CIRCULATION OF THE BLOOD

Matching

1.   D, p. 435
2.   B, p. 435
3.   C, p. 435
4.   G, p. 435
5.   A, p. 437
6.   E, p. 435
7.   F, p. 435

Matching

8.   I, p. 441
9.   B, p. 441
10.   D, p 441
11.   E, p. 441
12.   A, p. 441
13.   C, p. 441
14.   F, p. 442
15.   G, p. 444
16.   J, p. 444
17.   H, p. 441

Circle the Correct Answer

18.   D, p. 444

19.   C, p. 444
20.   B, p. 444
21.   B, p. 444
22.   D, p. 444
23.   B, p. 445
24.   B, p. 446
25.   A, p. 446
26.   D, p. 444

True or False

27.   F (Highest/arteries; lowest/veins), p. 448
28.   F (Blood pressure gradient), p. 448
29.   F (Stop), p. 448
30.   F (High blood pressure), p. 448
31.   F (Decreases), p. 448
32.   T
33.   T
34.   T
35.   F (Increases blood pressure/weaker heartbeat tends to decrease it), p. 451
36.   F (Contract), p. 451
37.   F (Relax), p. 451
38.   T
39.   T
40.   F (Right), p. 451
41.   F (Artery), p. 452
42.   T
43.   T
44.   F (Brachial), p. 452

Fill in the Blanks

45.   Septic shock, p. 454
46.   Cardiogenic shock, p. 453
47.   Anaphylaxis; anaphylactic shock, p. 453
48.   Neurogenic shock, p. 453
49.   Low blood volume, p. 453
50.   Toxic shock syndrome, p. 454

Unscramble the Words

51.   Systemic
52.   Venule
53.   Artery
54.   Pulse
55.   Vessel

Applying What You Know

56.   Anaphylactic shock
57.   Hypovolemic shock
58.   Varicose veins; wear support stockings
59.   Hemorrhage

60. WORD FIND

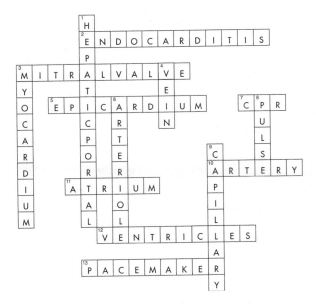

```
Y H Y  S I S O B M O R H T A  R
L A C I L I B M U O A Y N I  Y
E E S Y S T E M I C C G D E  U
M V E N U L E D D C I X M D  I
E Y M U I R T A R N L E C G  Y
N O I T A Z I R A L O P E D  N
U D L A T R O P C I T A P E  H
S I U K M U E T O E S L U P  U
R P N F Y C B E D R A L Z P  J
D S A H T I T V N L I B D W
Q U R O I V A Q E O D A K R  K
K C R M P G A I G N D D Z Y  J
Y I Y R I N E A F Z L Q S P  X
S R M I C C Q O A W U N H O  K
P T A V H H Z L H I J J X K  Z
```

Crossword

```
        ¹H
       ²E N D O C A R D I T I S
        P
³M I T R A L V A L V E⁴
Y       T           E
O   ⁵E P I C A R D I U M    ⁷C⁸P R
C       C       R       N       U
A       P       T               L
R       O       E       ⁹C       S
D       R       R   ¹⁰A R T E R Y
I   ¹¹A T R I U M       P
U       A       O       I
M       L       L       L
        ¹²V E N T R I C L E S
                        A
    ¹³P A C E M A K E R  Y
```

Check Your Knowledge

Multiple Choice

1. C, p. 441
2. A, p. 454
3. C, p. 453
4. C, p. 435
5. C, p. 436
6. B, p. 442
7. A, p. 445
8. A, p. 448
9. D, p. 441
10. B, p. 441

Matching

11. G, p. 435
12. A, p. 441
13. I, p. 442
14. C, p. 446
15. F, p. 441
16. B, p. 442
17. H, p. 444
18. D, p. 441
19. E, p. 435
20. J, p. 453

Fetal Circulation

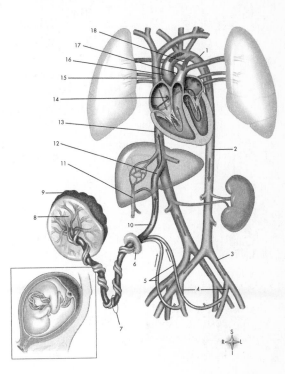

1. Aortic arch
2. Abdominal aorta
3. Common iliac artery
4. Internal iliac arteries
5. Umbilical arteries
6. Fetal umbilicus
7. Umbilical cord
8. Fetal side of placenta
9. Maternal side of placenta
10. Umbilical vein
11. Hepatic portal vein
12. Ductus venosus
13. Inferior vena cava
14. Foramen ovale
15. Superior vena cava
16. Ascending aorta
17. Pulmonary trunk
18. Ductus arteriosus

Hepatic Portal Circulation

Principal Arteries of the Body

1.   Inferior vena cava
2.   Stomach
3.   Gastric vein
4.   Spleen
5.   Pancreatic vein
6.   Splenic vein
7.   Gastroepiploic vein
8.   Descending colon
9.   Inferior mesenteric vein
10. Small intestine
11. Appendix
12. Ascending colon
13. Superior mesenteric vein
14. Pancreas
15. Duodenum
16. Hepatic portal vein
17. Liver
18. Hepatic veins

1.   Occipital
2.   Internal carotid
3.   External carotid
4.   Left common carotid
5.   Left subclavian
6.   Arch of aorta
7.   Pulmonary
8.   Left coronary
9.   Aorta
10. Celiac
11. Splenic
12. Renal
13. Inferior mesenteric
14. Radial
15. Ulnar
16. Anterior tibial
17. Popliteal
18. Femoral
19. Deep femoral
20. External iliac
21. Internal iliac
22. Common iliac
23. Abdominal aorta
24. Superior mesenteric
25. Brachial
26. Axillary
27. Right coronary
28. Brachiocephalic
29. Right common carotid
30. Facial

Principal Veins of the Body

1. Superior sagittal sinus
2. External jugular
3. Internal jugular
4. Left brachiocephalic
5. Left subclavian
6. Cephalic
7. Axillary
8. Great cardiac
9. Basilic
10. Long thoracic
11. Splenic
12. Inferior mesenteric
13. Common iliac
14. Internal iliac
15. Femoral
16. Popliteal
17. Peroneal
18. Anterior tibial
19. Posterior tibial
20. Great saphenous
21. Femoral
22. External iliac
23. Common iliac
24. Superior mesenteric
25. Median cubital
26. Hepatic portal
27. Hepatic
28. Inferior vena cava
29. Small cardiac
30. Pulmonary (right)

31. Superior vena cava
32. Right subclavian
33. Right brachiocephalic
34. Facial

CHAPTER 15
THE LYMPHATIC SYSTEM AND IMMUNITY

Fill in the Blanks

1. Lymph, p. 462
2. Interstitial fluid, p. 462
3. Lymphatic capillaries, p. 462
4. Right lymphatic duct and thoracic duct, p. 463
5. Cisterna chyli, p. 463
6. Lymph nodes, p. 464
7. Afferent, p. 464
8. Efferent, p. 464
9. Lymphedema, p. 464
10. Lymphoma, p. 466

Choose the Correct Response

11. B, p. 467
12. C, p. 468
13. C, p. 468
14. A, p. 467
15. C, p. 468
16. A, p. 467
17. A, p. 467

Matching

18. C, p. 468
19. A, p. 469
20. E, p. 469
21. B, p. 469
22. D, p. 469

Matching

23. C, p. 474
24. A, p. 470
25. F, p. 470
26. B, p. 470
27. G, p. 470
28. D, p. 471
29. H, p. 474
30. E, p. 472

Multiple Choice

31. D, p. 473
32. D, p. 474
33. C, p. 475

34. C, p. 474
35. C, p. 474
36. E, p. 476
37. E, p. 476
38. C, p. 476
39. E, p. 476
40. E, p. 476
41. A, p. 476
42. B, p. 476

Circle the Correct Answer

43. Hypersensitivity, p. 477
44. Allergens, p. 477
45. Anaphylactic shock, p. 477
46. Lupus, p. 478
47. Isoimmunity, p. 478
48. HLAs, p. 479

Select the Correct Response

49. B, p. 481
50. A, p. 480
51. A, p. 480
52. B, p. 480
53. A, p. 480

Unscramble the Words

54. Complement
55. Immunity
56. Clones
57. Interferon
58. Memory cells

Applying What You Know

59. Natural active immunity
60. AIDS
61. Baby Wilson had no means of producing T cells, thus making him susceptible to several diseases. Isolation was a means of controlling his exposure to these diseases.

62. **WORD FIND**

Crossword

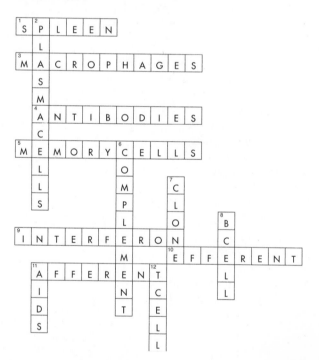

Check Your Knowledge

Multiple Choice

1. A, p. 467
2. A, p. 462
3. D, p. 481
4. B, p. 479
5. D, p. 474
6. B, p. 472
7. D, p. 472
8. D, p. 472
9. D, p. 474
10. C, p. 470

Matching

11. E, p. 467
12. D, p. 476
13. I, p. 474
14. H, p. 481
15. G, p. 472
16. B, p. 464
17. A, p. 463
18. J, p. 476
19. C, p. 470
20. F, p. 470

Principal Organs of the Lymphatic System

1. Cervical lymph nodes
2. Submandibular nodes
3. Thymus
4. Axillary lymph nodes
5. Thoracic duct
6. Spleen
7. Cisterna chyli
8. Inguinal lymph nodes
9. Popliteal lymph nodes
10. Lymph vessels
11. Red bone marrow
12. Right lymphatic duct

CHAPTER 16
THE RESPIRATORY SYSTEM

Matching

1. J, p. 490
2. G, p. 490
3. A, p. 490
4. I, p. 493
5. B, p. 492
6. F, p. 492
7. C, p. 493
8. H, p. 490
9. D, p. 490
10. E, p. 490

Fill in the Blanks

11. Air distributor, p. 490
12. Gas exchanger, p. 490
13. Filters, p. 490
14. Warms, p. 490
15. Humidifies, p. 490
16. Nose, p. 490
17. Pharynx, p. 490
18. Larynx, p. 490
19. Trachea, p. 490
20. Bronchi, p. 490
21. Lungs, p. 490
22. Alveoli, p. 490
23. Diffusion, p. 490
24. Respiratory membrane, p. 490
25. Surface, p. 490

Circle the One That Does Not Belong

26. Oropharynx (the others refer to the nose)
27. Conchae (the others refer to paranasal sinuses)
28. Epiglottis (the others refer to the pharynx)
29. Uvula (the others refer to the adenoids)
30. Larynx (the others refer to the eustachian tubes)
31. Tonsils (the others refer to the larynx)
32. Eustachian tube (the others refer to the tonsils)
33. Pharynx (the others refer to the larynx)

Choose the Correct Response

34. A, p. 495
35. B, p. 495
36. A, p. 493
37. A, p. 495
38. A, p. 493
39. B, p. 495
40. B, p. 495
41. C, p. 497
42. A, p. 498

43. B, p. 498
44. A, p. 500

Fill in the Blanks

45. Trachea, p. 500
46. C-rings of cartilage, p. 500
47. Heimlich maneuver, p. 501
48. Primary bronchi, p. 501
49. Alveolar sacs, p. 501
50. Apex, p. 503
51. Pleura, p. 503
52. Pleurisy, p. 503
53. Pneumothorax, p. 503

True or False

54. F (Breathing), p. 506
55. F (Expiration), p. 506
56. F (Down), p. 507
57. F (Internal respiration), p. 506
58. T
59. F (1 pint), p. 510
60. T
61. F (Vital capacity), p. 510
62. T

Multiple Choice

63. E, p. 506
64. C, p. 507
65. C, p. 507
66. B, p. 506
67. D, p. 510
68. D, p. 510
69. D, p. 510

Matching

70. E, p. 512
71. B, p. 512
72. G, p. 512
73. A, p. 513
74. F, p. 513
75. D, p. 512
76. C, p. 512

Fill in the Blanks

77. Pneumonia, p. 514
78. Tuberculosis, p. 514
79. Emphysema, p. 516
80. Asthma, p. 516

Unscramble the Words

81. Pleurisy
82. Bronchitis
83. Epistaxis

84. Adenoids
85. Inspiration

Applying What You Know

86. During the day, Mr. Gorski's cilia are paralyzed because of his heavy smoking. They use the time when Mr. Gorski is asleep to sweep accumulations of mucus and bacteria toward the pharynx. When Mr. Gorski awakens, these collections are waiting to be eliminated.
87. Impossible for air to travel from the nose into the throat. The individual may be forced to breathe through the mouth.
88. During expiration, the alveoli are unable to force out a normal amount of air. Residual volume is increased at the expense of the expiratory reserve volume. Pulmonary infections can cause inflammation and an accumulation of fluid in the air spaces of the lungs. The fluid reduces the amount of space available for air and thus decreases the vital capacity.

89. **WORD FIND**

Crossword

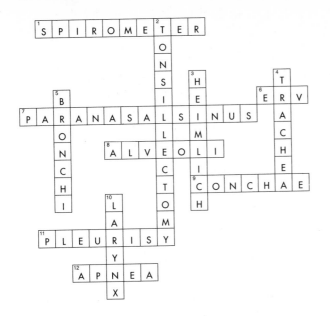

Sagittal View of Face and Neck

Check Your Knowledge

Multiple Choice

1. A, p. 512
2. B, p. 495
3. D, p. 503
4. B, p. 510
5. A, p. 503
6. D, p. 497
7. A, p. 500
8. C, p. 507
9. D, p. 506
10. B, p. 495

Matching

11. E, p. 497
12. I, p. 506
13. A, p. 503
14. G, p. 503
15. D, p. 508
16. B, p. 495
17. C, p. 493
18. H, p. 501
19. F, p. 490
20. J, p. 503

1. Sphenoidal air sinus
2. Pharyngeal tonsil (adenoids)
3. Opening of auditory (eustachian) tube
4. Nasopharynx
5. Soft palate
6. Uvula
7. Palatine tonsil
8. Oropharynx
9. Epiglottis
10. Laryngopharynx
11. Esophagus
12. Trachea
13. Vocal cords
14. Thyroid cartilage
15. Hyoid bone
16. Lingual tonsil
17. Hard palate
18. Inferior concha
19. Middle concha
20. Superior concha
21. Nasal bone
22. Frontal air sinus

Respiratory Organs

1. Nasal cavity
2. Nasopharynx
3. Oropharynx
4. Laryngopharynx
5. Larynx
6. Pharynx
7. Trachea
8. Bronchioles
9. Left and right primary bronchi
10. Alveolar duct
11. Alveolar sac
12. Capillary
13. Alveoli

Pulmonary Ventilation Volumes

1. Total lung capacity
2. Inspiratory reserve volume
3. Tidal volume
4. Expiratory reserve volume
5. Residual volume

CHAPTER 17
THE DIGESTIVE SYSTEM

Fill in the Blanks

1. Gastrointestinal tract or G.I. tract, p. 527
2. Mechanical, p. 528
3. Chemical, p. 528
4. Feces, p. 528
5. Digestion, absorption, and metabolism, p. 528

Select the Correct Response

6. A, p. 529
7. B, p. 529
8. B, p. 529
9. A, p. 529
10. A, p. 529
11. A, p. 529
12. A, p. 529
13. A, p. 529
14. B, p. 529
15. B, p. 529
16. B, p. 529
17. B, p. 529

Multiple Choice

18. E, p. 529
19. C, p. 530
20. E, p. 530
21. D, p. 530
22. B, p. 532
23. C, p. 531
24. D, p. 531
25. D, p. 531
26. D, p. 533
27. A, p. 535
28. C, p. 535
29. A, p. 535
30. A, P. 530
31. B, p. 531
32. C, p. 530

Fill in the Blanks

33. Visceral peritoneum, p. 536
34. Mouth; anus, p. 536
35. Lumen, p. 536
36. Mucosa, p. 536
37. Submucosa, p. 536
38. Peristalsis, p. 536
39. Serosa, p. 536
40. Mesentery, p. 536

Fill in the Blanks

41. Pharynx, p. 535
42. Esophagus, p. 536
43. Stomach, p. 536
44. Lower esophageal sphincter, p. 536
45. Chyme, p. 539
46. Fundus, p. 540
47. Body, p. 540
48. Pylorus, p. 540
49. Pyloric sphincter, p. 540
50. Small intestine, p. 540

Matching

51. D, p. 540
52. J, p. 540
53. G, p. 536
54. A, p. 536
55. H, p. 541
56. B, p. 539
57. C, p. 540
58. E, p. 541
59. I, p. 537
60. F, p. 540

Multiple Choice

61. C, p. 542
62. B, p. 542
63. A, p. 545
64. A, p. 545
65. B, p. 542
66. E, p. 542
67. D, p. 545
68. D, p. 545
69. B, p. 545
70. C, p. 545

True or False

71. F (Vitamin K), p. 548
72. F (No villi are present in the large intestine), p. 548
73. F (Diarrhea), p. 550
74. F (Cecum), p. 549
75. F (Hepatic), p. 549
76. F (Sigmoid), p. 549
77. T
78. T
79. F (Parietal), p. 553
80. F (Mesentery), p. 553
81. F (Diverticulitis), p. 550
82. T
83. T
84. F (Ascites), p. 553

Multiple Choice

85. B, p. 554
86. D, p. 554
87. C, p. 554
88. C, p. 554
89. C, p. 554

Chemical Digestion

90. Fill in the blank areas on the chart below.

DIGESTIVE JUICES AND ENZYMES	SUBSTANCE DIGESTED (OR HYDROLYZED)	RESULTING PRODUCT
Saliva		
1.	1. Starch (polysaccharide)	1.
Gastric Juice		
2.	2.	2. Partially digested proteins
Pancreatic Juice		
3.	3.	3. Peptides and amino acids
4.	4. Fats emulsified by bile	4.
5.	5. Starch	5.
Intestinal Enzymes		
6.	6. Peptides	6.
7. Sucrase	7.	7.
8.	8. Lactose	8.
9.	9.	9. Glucose

Unscramble the Words

91. Bolus
92. Chyme
93. Papilla
94. Peritoneum
95. Lace apron

Applying What You Know

96. Ulcer
97. Pylorospasm
98. Cholelithiasis; cholecystectomy

99. **WORD FIND**

Check Your Knowledge

Multiple Choice

1. A, p. 545
2. C, p. 539
3. A, p. 542
4. B, p. 530
5. B, p. 536
6. B, p. 542
7. B, p. 553
8. C, p. 554
9. C, p. 554
10. A, p. 554

Completion

11. N, p. 549
12. J, p. 553
13. P, p. 554
14. Q, R, A, p. 542
15. W, p. 545
16. H, K, D, p. 528
17. E, p. 545
18. T, U, C, X, p. 536
19. G, p. 536
20. I, O, S, F, p. 530

Crossword

Location of Digestive Organs

Tooth

1. Vermiform appendix
2. Region of ileocecal valve
3. Cecum
4. Ileum
5. Ascending colon
6. Transverse colon
7. Hepatic flexure
8. Liver
9. Diaphragm
10. Esophagus
11. Trachea
12. Pharynx
13. Submandibular gland
14. Parotid gland
15. Tongue
16. Sublingual gland
17. Larynx
18. Spleen
19. Splenic flexure
20. Stomach
21. Descending colon
22. Sigmoid colon
23. Rectum
24. Anal canal
25. Hepatic bile duct
26. Liver
27. Cystic duct
28. Gallbladder
29. Duodenum
30. Pancreas
31. Spleen

1. Cusp
2. Enamel
3. Dentin
4. Pulp cavity with nerves and vessels
5. Gingiva (gum)
6. Root canal
7. Periodontal ligament
8. Periodontal membrane
9. Cementum
10. Bone
11. Root
12. Neck
13. Crown

The Salivary Glands

1. Parotid gland
2. Parotid duct
3. Submandibular gland
4. Submandibular duct
5. Sublingual gland

Stomach

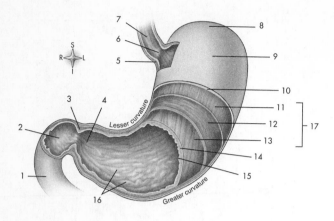

Gallbladder and Bile Ducts

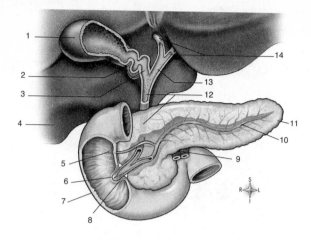

1.	Duodenum
2.	Duodenal bulb
3.	Pyloric sphincter
4.	Pylorus
5.	Lower esophageal sphincter
6.	Gastroesophageal sphincter
7.	Esophagus
8.	Fundus
9.	Body of stomach
10.	Serosa
11.	Longitudinal muscle layer
12.	Circular muscle layer
13.	Oblique muscle layer
14.	Submucosa
15.	Mucosa
16.	Rugae
17.	Muscularis

1.	Corpus (body) of gallbladder
2.	Neck of gallbladder
3.	Cystic duct
4.	Liver
5.	Lesser duodenal papilla
6.	Greater duodenal papilla
7.	Duodenum
8.	Sphincter muscles
9.	Superior mesenteric artery and vein
10.	Pancreatic duct
11.	Pancreas
12.	Common bile duct
13.	Common hepatic duct
14.	Right and left hepatic ducts

The Small Intestine

Segment
of jejunum

Magnification
of jejunal
mucosal wall

Villi epithelium

Mucosa villi

1.   Mesentery
2.   Longitudinal muscle
3.   Circular muscle
4.   Submucosa
5.   Mucosa
6.   Plica (fold)
7.   Lymph node
8.   Mucosa
9.   Single villus
10.   Epithelium
11.   Microvilli
12.   Mucosa
13.   Vein
14.   Artery
15.   Lacteal (lymph)
16.   Microvilli
17.   Epithelial cell

The Large Intestine

1.   Aorta
2.   Splenic vein
3.   Superior mesenteric artery
4.   Splenic (left colic) flexure
5.   Inferior mesenteric artery and vein
6.   Descending colon
7.   Sigmoid colon
8.   Rectum
9.   Mesentery
10.   Ileum
11.   Vermiform appendix
12.   Cecum
13.   Ileocecal valve
14.   Ascending colon
15.   Hepatic (right colic) flexure
16.   Transverse colon
17.   Inferior vena cava
18.   Portal vein

CHAPTER 18
NUTRITION AND METABOLISM

Fill in the Blanks

1. Bile, p. 567
2. Prothrombin, p. 568
3. Fibrinogen, p. 568
4. Iron, p. 568
5. Hepatic portal vein, p. 568

Matching

6. B, p. 570
7. A, p. 568
8. C, p. 571
9. D, p. 572
10. E, p. 574
11. A, p. 568
12. E, p. 574
13. A, p. 568

Circle the Word that Does Not Belong

14. Bile (all others refer to carbohydrate metabolism)
15. Amino acids (all others refer to fat metabolism)
16. M (all others refer to vitamins)
17. Iron (all others refer to protein metabolism)
18. Insulin (all others tend to increase blood glucose)
19. Folic acid (all others are minerals)
20. Ascorbic acid (all others refer to the B-complex vitamins)

Multiple Choice

21. C, p. 574
22. A, p. 574
23. A, p. 576
24. D, p. 576
25. D, p. 576

Choose the Correct Response

26. B, p. 570
27. C, p. 576
28. G, p. 577
29. F, p. 576
30. A, p. 575
31. H, p. 577
32. E, p. 576
33. D, p. 576

Multiple Choice

34. C, p. 578

35. B, p. 578
36. B, p. 578
37. A, p. 578
38. C, p. 578
39. D, p. 578

True or False

40. T
41. F (Hypothermia), p. 580
42. T
43. F (Heat stroke), p. 580
44. F (Malignant hyperthermia), p. 579

Unscramble the Words

45. Liver
46. Catabolism
47. Amino
48. Pyruvic
49. Evaporation

Applying What You Know

50. Weight loss and anorexia nervosa
51. Iron; meat, eggs, vegetables, and legumes
52. He was carbohydrate loading or glycogen loading, which allows the muscles to sustain aerobic exercise for up to 50% longer than usual.

53. **WORD FIND**

Crossword

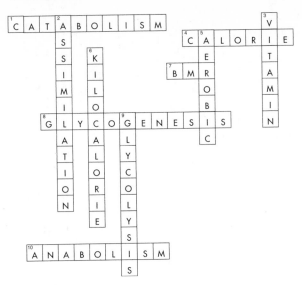

Check Your Knowledge

Multiple Choice

1. B, p. 568
2. A, p. 568
3. C, p. 570
4. C, p. 574
5. B, p. 574
6. B, p. 570
7. A, p. 570
8. A, p. 578
9. B, p. 567
10. D, p. 568

Completion

11. C, D, I, p. 567
12. E, p. 568
13. J, p. 568
14. G, p. 568
15. B, p. 570
16. D, p. 571
17. L, p. 569
18. A, p. 572
19. K, H, p. 574
20. F, p. 568

CHAPTER 19
THE URINARY SYSTEM

Multiple Choice

1. E, p. 591
2. C, p. 592
3. E, p. 592
4. C, p. 594
5. E, p. 596
6. C, p. 596
7. B, p. 596
8. E, p. 596
9. C, p. 596
10. C, p. 597
11. B, p. 597 (Review Chapter 11)
12. D, p. 597

Choose the Correct Term

13. G, p. 592
14. I, p. 595
15. H, p. 595
16. B, p. 591
17. K, p. 592
18. F, p. 592
19. J, p. 592
20. D, p. 592
21. L, p. 592
22. C, p. 592
23. E, p. 592
24. A, p. 592

Choose the Correct Term

25. C, p. 599
26. B, p. 599
27. C, p. 599
28. A, p. 598
29. B, p. 599
30. C, p. 599
31. C, p. 599
32. A, p. 598
33. C, p. 600 Figure 19-7
34. B, p. 599
35. A, p. 598
36. B, p. 599

Fill in the Blanks

37. Urinalysis, p. 598
38. Mucous membrane, p. 598
39. Centrifuge, p. 599
40. Anuria, p. 598
41. Cystitis or bladder infections, p. 601
42. Semen, p. 599
43. Urinary meatus, p. 599

Fill in the Blanks

44. Micturition, p. 600
45. Urination, p. 600
46. Voiding, p. 600
47. Internal urethral sphincter, p. 600
48. Exit, p. 600

49. Urethra, p. 600
50. Voluntary, p. 601
51. Emptying reflex, p. 601
52. Urethra, p. 601
53. Retention, p. 601
54. Suppression, p. 601
55. Stress incontinence, p. 601

Select the Correct Answer

56. I, p. 602
57. C, p. 602
58. G, p. 601
59. F, p. 603
60. K, p. 603
61. A, p. 604
62. H, p. 605
63. J, p. 605
64. B, p. 602
65. D, p. 605
66. E, p. 605
67. L, p. 603

Unscramble the Words

68. Calyx
69. Voiding
70. Papilla
71. Glomerulus
72. Pyramids

Applying What You Know

73. Polyuria
74. Residual urine is often the cause of repeated cystitis.
75. A high percentage of catheterized patients develop cystitis, often due to poor aseptic technique when inserting the catheter.
76. Hemorrhage causes a drop in blood pressure, which decreases the urine output and can eventually lead to kidney failure.

77. **WORD FIND**

Crossword

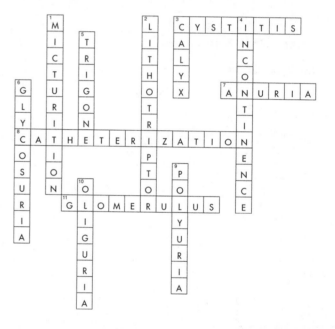

Check Your Knowledge

Multiple Choice

1. D, p. 601
2. B, p. 606
3. D, p. 589
4. A, p. 597
5. C, p. 601
6. C, p. 596
7. B, p. 601
8. C, p. 598
9. B, p. 592
10. A, p. 592

Matching

11.   E, p. 601
12.   C, p. 598
13.   F, p. 603
14.   D, p. 600
15.   J, p. 598
16.   H, p. 598
17.   A, p. 601
18.   G, p. 603
19.   I, p. 601
20.   B, p. 596

Urinary System

1.   Spleen
2.   Renal artery
3.   Renal vein
4.   Left kidney
5.   Inferior vena cava
6.   Abdominal aorta
7.   Common iliac vein
8.   Common iliac artery
9.   Urethra
10.   Urinary bladder
11.   Ureter
12.   Right kidney
13.   Tenth rib
14.   Liver
15.   Adrenal glands

Kidney

1.   Interlobular arteries
2.   Renal column
3.   Renal sinus
4.   Hilum
5.   Renal pelvis
6.   Renal papilla of pyramid
7.   Ureter
8.   Medulla
9.   Medullary pyramid
10.   Major calyces
11.   Minor calyces
12.   Cortex
13.   Capsule

Nephron

1. Proximal convoluted tubule
2. Collecting tubule
3. Descending limb of Henle's loop
4. Ascending limb of Henle's loop
5. Descending limb of Henle's loop
6. Artery and vein
7. Distal convoluted tubule
8. Peritubular capillaries
9. Afferent arteriole
10. Juxtaglomerular apparatus
11. Efferent arteriole
12. Glomerulus
13. Bowman's capsule

CHAPTER 20
FLUID AND ELECTROLYTE BALANCE

Circle the Correct Answer

1. Inside, p. 619
2. Extracellular, p. 619
3. Extracellular, p. 619
4. Lower, p. 618
5. More, p. 618
6. Decline, p. 619
7. Less, p. 618
8. Decreases, p. 619
9. 55%, p. 618
10. Fluid balance, p. 617

Multiple Choice

11. A, p. 622
12. D, p. 622
13. A, p. 622
14. C, p. 621
15. E, p. 621
16. D, p. 621
17. D, p. 623
18. C, p. 623
19. B, p. 623
20. D, p. 626
21. E, p. 625
22. B, p. 625
23. B, p. 626
24. B, p. 626

True or False

25. F (Catabolism), p. 621
26. T
27. T
28. F (Nonelectrolyte), p. 621
29. T
30. F (Hypervolemia), p. 624, Figure 20-6
31. F (Tubular function), p. 626
32. F (2400 ml), p. 621
33. T
34. F (100 mEq), p. 623

Fill in the Blanks

35. Dehydration, p. 626
36. Decreases, p. 626
37. Decrease, p. 626
38. Overhydration, p. 626
39. Intravenous fluids, p. 626
40. Heart, p. 626
41. Hypernatremia, p. 626
42. Hyperkalemia, p. 626

Applying What You Know

43. Ms. Titus could not accurately measure water intake created by foods or catabolism, nor could she measure output created by lungs, skin, or the intestines.
44. A careful record of fluid intake and output should be maintained, and the patient should be monitored for signs and symptoms of electrolyte and water imbalance.
45. Jack's body contained more water. Obese people have a lower water content than slender people.

46. WORD FIND

Crossword

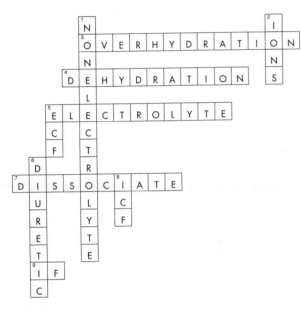

Check Your Knowledge

Multiple Choice

1. A, p. 618
2. D, p. 620
3. D, p. 626
4. C, p. 626
5. A, p. 623
6. B, p. 624
7. D, p. 620
8. A, p. 624
9. A, p. 621
10. D, p. 624

Completion

11. E, p. 626
12. B, p. 624
13. J, M, K, p. 619
14. F, p. 622
15. D, p. 624
16. L, p. 621
17. I, p. 626
18. C, p. 626
19. H and A, p. 621
20. N, p. 617

CHAPTER 21
ACID-BASE BALANCE

Choose the Correct Term

1. B, p. 636
2. A, p. 636
3. A, p. 636
4 B, p. 636
5. B, p. 636
6. B, p. 636
7. B, p. 636
8. A, p. 636
9. B, p. 636
10. B, p. 636

Multiple Choice

11. E, p. 636
12. E, p. 637
13. A, p. 637
14. E, p. 639
15. C, p. 639
16. D, p. 639
17. C, p. 640
18. B, p. 640
19. D, p. 641
20. E, p. 641
21. E, p. 641

True or False

22. F (Buffer instead of heart), p. 636
23. F (Buffer pairs), p. 637
24. T
25. T
26. F (Alkalosis), p. 640
27. F (Reverse—arterial blood has a higher pH), p. 636
28. T
29. F (Kidneys), p. 644
30. F (Lungs), p. 644

Matching

31.   E, p. 643
32.   G, p. 645
33.   F, p. 643
34.   A, p. 645
35.   I, p. 643
36.   B, p. 645
37.   H, p. 645
38.   C, p. 645
39.   D, p. 645
40.   J, p. 643

Applying What You Know

41.   Normal saline contains chloride ions, which replace bicarbonate ions and thus relieve the bicarbonate excess that occurs during severe vomiting.
42.   Most citrus fruits, although acid-tasting, are fully oxidized with the help of buffers during metabolism and have little effect on acid-base balance. Cranberry juice is one of the few exceptions.
43.   Milk of magnesia. It is a base. Interestingly, milk is slightly acidic.

44.   **WORD FIND**

Crossword

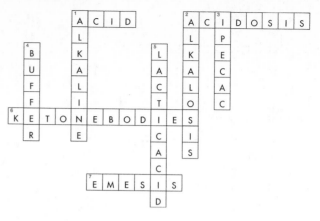

Check Your Knowledge

Multiple Choice

1.   A, p. 637
2.   C, p. 637
3.   A, p. 640
4.   D, p. 636
5.   A, p. 645
6.   D, p. 645
7.   D, p. 638
8.   D, p. 643
9.   D, p. 637
10.   A, p. 638

Matching

11.   G, p. 636
12.   C, p. 636
13.   I, p. 637
14.   E, p. 645
15.   F, p. 645
16.   A, p. 645
17.   B, p. 645
18.   D, p. 638
19.   J, p. 640
20.   H, p. 645

CHAPTER 22
THE REPRODUCTIVE SYSTEMS

Matching

Group A

1.   D, p. 654
2.   C, p. 654
3.   E, p. 653
4.   B, p. 655
5.   A, p. 653

Group B

6. C, p. 655
7. A, p. 655
8. D, p. 653
9. B, p. 655
10. E, p. 655

Multiple Choice

11. B, p. 655
12. C, p. 657
13. A, p. 657
14. D, p. 655
15. E, p. 657
16. D, p. 657
17. C, p. 659
18. C, p. 657
19. A, p. 657

Fill in the Blanks

20. Testes, p. 655
21. Spermatozoa or sperm, p. 657
22. Ovum, p. 654
23. Testosterone, p. 659
24. Interstitial cells, p. 659
25. Masculinizing, p. 659
26. Anabolic, p. 659

Choose the Correct Term

27. B, p. 660
28. H, p. 661
29. G, p. 660
30. A, p. 660
31. F, p. 660
32. C, p. 660
33. I, p. 660
34. E, p. 660
35. D, p. 662
36. J, p. 661

Fill in the Blanks

37. Oligospermia, p. 662
38. 2 months, p. 662
39. Cryptorchidism, p. 662
40. Benign prostatic hypertrophy, p. 663
41. Phimosis, p. 662
42. Impotence, p. 664
43. Hydrocele, p. 664
44. Inguinal hernia, p. 664
45. Prostate, p. 663

Matching

46. D, p. 665

47. C, p. 665
48. B, p. 665
49. A, p. 665
50. E, p. 667

Choose the Correct Structure

51. A, p. 671
52. B, p. 669
53. A, p. 671
54. B, p. 671
55. A, p. 671
56. A, p. 671
57. A, p. 671
58. B, p. 669

Fill in the Blanks

59. Gonads, p. 665
60. Oogenesis, p. 667
61. Meiosis, p. 667
62. One-half (or 23), p. 667
63. Fertilization, p. 667
64. 46, p. 667
65. Estrogen, p. 667
66. Progesterone, p. 667
67. Secondary sexual characteristics, p. 667
68. Menstrual cycle, p. 667
69. Puberty, p. 667

Choose the Correct Structure

70. A, p. 669
71. B, p. 668
72. C, p. 669
73. B, p. 668
74. A, p. 668
75. B, p. 668
76. A, p. 668
77. A, p. 668
78. C, p. 669

Matching

Group A

79. D, p. 670
80. E, p. 670
81. B, p. 670
82. C, p. 670
83. A, p. 670

Group B

84. E, p. 670
85. A, p. 670
86. D, p. 672
87. B, p. 672
88. C, p. 672

334   Answers to Exercises

True or False

89.   F (Menarche), p. 672
90.   F (One), p. 672
91.   F (14), p. 672
92.   F (Menstrual period), p. 672
93.   T
94.   F (Anterior), p. 672

Choose the Correct Hormone

95.   B, p. 673
96.   A, p. 672
97.   B, p. 673
98.   B, p. 673
99.   A, p. 675

Choose the Correct Response

100.   F, p. 677
101.   E, p. 677
102.   A, p. 681
103.   H, p. 676
104.   I, p. 670
105.   G, p. 676
106.   C, p. 676
107.   B, p. 675
108.   L, p. 681
109.   D, p. 676
110.   J, p. 679
111.   K, p. 681

Applying What You Know

112.   Yes. The testes are not only essential organs of reproduction, but are also responsible for the "masculinizing" hormone. Without this hormone, Mr. Belinki will have no desire to reproduce.

113.   Sterile. The sperm count may be too low to reproduce but the remaining testicle will produce enough masculinizing hormone to prevent impotency.

114.   The uterine tubes are not attached to the ovaries and infections can exit at this area and enter the abdominal cavity.

115.   Yes. Without the hormones from the ovaries to initiate the menstrual cycle, Mrs. Harlan will no longer have a menstrual cycle and can be considered to be in menopause (cessation of menstrual cycle).

116.   No. Mrs. Kelly still will have her ovaries, which are the source of her hormones. She will not experience menopause due to this procedure.

117.   **WORD FIND**

Crossword

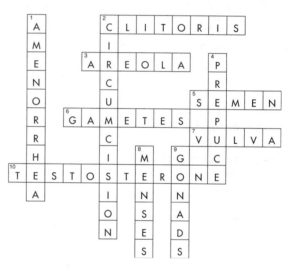

Check Your Knowledge

Multiple Choice

1.   A, p. 672
2.   D, p. 674
3.   D, p. 660
4.   C, p. 662
5.   C, p. 665
6.   A, p. 654
7.   B, p. 655
8.   C, p. 661
9.   A, p. 670
10.   D, p. 674

Completion

11.   C, p. 669
12.   L, p. 657

13. H, p. 660
14. G, p. 668
15. F, p. 660
16. K, p. 662
17. B, p. 668
18. D, p. 667
19. J, p. 672
20. I, p. 672

Tubules of Testis and Epididymis

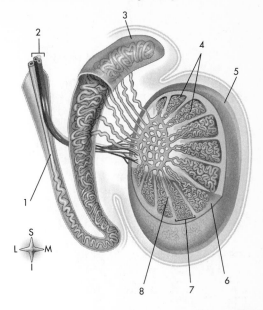

1. Ductus (vas) deferens
2. Nerves and blood vessels in the spermatic cord
3. Epididymis
4. Seminiferous tubules
5. Testis
6. Tunica albuginea
7. Lobule
8. Septum

Male Reproductive Organs

1. Seminal vesicle
2. Ejaculatory duct
3. Prostate gland
4. Rectum
5. Bulbourethral (Cowper's) gland
6. Anus
7. Scrotum
8. Testis
9. Epididymis
10. Penis
11. Urethra
12. Ductus deferens
13. Urinary bladder
14. Ureter

Vulva

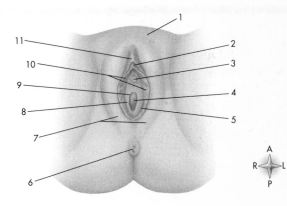

1. Mons pubis
2. Clitoris
3. Orifice of urethra
4. Orifice of vagina
5. Opening of greater vestibular gland
6. Anus
7. Labia majora
8. Vestibule
9. Hymen
10. Labia minora
11. Prepuce

Breast

Female Pelvis

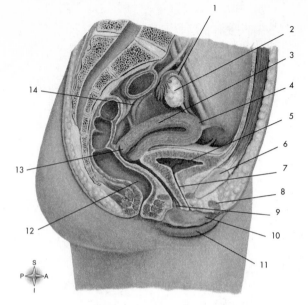

1.   Clavicle
2.   Pectoralis major muscle
3.   Intercostal muscles
4.   Nipple
5.   Lactiferous duct
6.   Alveoli
7.   Suspensory ligaments of Cooper

1.   Uterine (fallopian) tube
2.   Ovary
3.   Body of uterus
4.   Fundus of uterus
5.   Urinary bladder
6.   Symphysis pubis
7.   Urethra
8.   Clitoris
9.   Vagina
10. Labium minus
11. Labium majus
12. Rectum
13. Cervix
14. Ureter

Uterus and Adjacent Structures

1. Fundus
2. Body of uterus
3. Cervix
4. Vagina
5. Cervical canal
6. Perimetrium
7. Myometrium
8. Endometrium
9. Ovary
10. Fimbriae
11. Uterine (fallopian) tube

CHAPTER 23
GROWTH AND DEVELOPMENT

Fill in the Blanks

1. Conception, p. 692
2. Birth, p. 692
3. Embryology, p. 692
4. Oviduct, fallopian tube, or uterine tube, p. 692
5. Zygote, p. 692
6. Morula, p. 692
7. Blastocyst, p. 692
8. Amniotic cavity, p. 694
9. Chorion, p. 695
10. Placenta, p. 695

Choose the Correct Term

11. G, p. 693
12. F, p. 697
13. C, p. 705
14. B, p. 697
15. A, p. 693
16. H, p. 701
17. E, p. 701
18. D, p. 699
19. I, p. 697
20. J, p. 705

True or False

21. T
22. T
23. F (Placenta previa), p. 703
24. F (Abruptio placentae), p. 704
25. F (Preeclampsia), p. 704
26. F (Stillbirth), p. 705
27. T

Multiple Choice

28. E, p. 706
29. E, p. 707
30. E, p. 708
31. A, p. 708
32. B, p. 708
33. C, p. 708
34. B, p. 708
35. D, p. 708
36. E, p. 708
37. D, p. 709
38. A, p. 709
39. C, p. 709
40. C, p. 709
41. C, p. 709
42. E, p. 709

Matching

43. F, p. 706
44. A, p. 707
45. C, p. 709
46. H, p. 708
47. D, p. 709
48. B, p. 707
49. E, p. 709
50. G, p. 710
51. I, p. 710

Fill in the Blanks

52. Lipping, p. 710
53. Osteoarthritis, p. 710
54. Nephron, p. 710
55. Barrel chest, p. 712
56. Atherosclerosis, p. 713
57. Arteriosclerosis, p. 713
58. Hypertension, p. 713
59. Presbyopia, p. 713
60. Cataract, p. 713
61. Glaucoma, p. 713

Unscramble the Words

62. Infancy
63. Postnatal
64. Organogenesis

65. Zygote
66. Childhood
67. Fertilization

Applying What You Know

68. Normal
69. Only about 40% of the taste buds present at age 30 remain at age 75.
70. A significant loss of hair cells in the organ of Corti causes a serious decline in ability to hear certain frequencies.
71. Each baby girl had her own placenta.

72. **WORD FIND**

Crossword

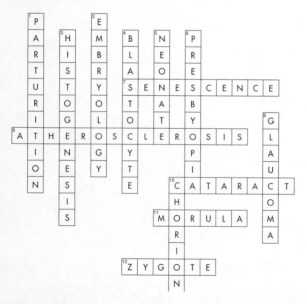

Check Your Knowledge

Multiple Choice

1. C, p. 692

2. D, p. 710
3. D, p. 709
4. A, p. 707
5. D, p. 713
6. D, p. 713
7. A, p. 714
8. A, p. 709
9. C, p. 709
10. B, p. 697

Matching

11. E, p. 713
12. G, p. 713
13. C, p. 701
14. I, p. 713
15. H, p. 709
16. D, p. 695
17. J, p. 713
18. F, p. 710
19. A, p. 713
20. B, p. 695

Fertilization and Implantation

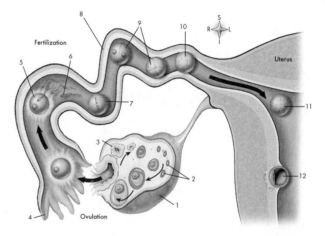

1. Ovary
2. Developing follicles
3. Corpus luteum
4. Fimbriae
5. Discharged ovum
6. Spermatozoa
7. First mitosis
8. Uterine (fallopian) tube
9. Divided zygote
10. Morula
11. Blastocyst
12. Implantation

CHAPTER 24
GENETICS AND GENETIC DISEASES

Matching

1. E, p. 724
2. A, p. 724
3. B, p. 726
4. C, p. 726
5. D, p. 726
6. G, p. 724
7. I, p. 724
8. J, p. 726
9. H, p. 726
10. F, p. 726

Fill in the Blanks

11. Genes, p. 726
12. Dominant, p. 728
13. Recessive, p. 728
14. Carrier, p. 728
15. Co-dominance, p. 728
16. Sex, p. 728
17. Female, p. 728
18. Mutation, p. 730
19. Genetic mutation, p. 730

Matching

20. E, p. 732
21. D, p. 731
22. J, p. 732
23. F, p. 734
24. C, p. 732
25. G, p. 735
26. A, p. 732
27. H, p. 735
28. B, p. 732
29. I, p. 736

Multiple Choice

30. D, p. 736
31. B, p. 736
32. C, p. 738
33. C, p. 736
34. D, p. 738
35. D, p. 740
36. B, p. 739

True or False

37. T
38. F (Electrophoresis), p. 740
39. F (Gene augmentation), p. 739
40. T
41. T

Unscramble the Words

42. Carrier
43. Trisomy
44. Gene
45. Pedigree
46. Chromosome
47. Inherited

Applying What You Know

48. In a form of dominance called *co-dominance*, the effect will be equal, causing "light brown" to occur.
49. One in four or 25%
50. Amniocentesis or chorionic villus sampling. The counselor will then produce a karyotype to determine anomalies.

51. **PUNNETT SQUARE**
Mr. Fortner PP
Mrs. Fortner pp
a. 100% chance of brown eyes and 0% chance of blue eyes
b. Yes
c. 25%
Mrs. Harrington Pp
Mr. Harrington Pp
a. Normal pigmentation 25%
b. Carriers 50%
c. Albinism 25%

52. **WORD FIND**

Crossword

Completion

11.   H, p. 738
12.   K, p. 738
13.   C, p. 734
14.   E, p. 724 (Review Chapter 3)
15.   A, p. 732
16.   G, p. 736
17.   D, p. 728
18.   J, p. 734
19.   L, p. 734
20.   B, p. 735

Check Your Knowledge

Multiple Choice

1.   A, p. 726
2.   D, p. 736
3.   C, p. 728
4.   B, p. 726
5.   A, p. 726
6.   C, p. 724
7.   B, p. 729
8.   C, p. 728
9.   A, p. 736
10.   B, p. 736